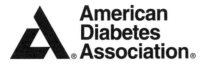

American Diabetes Association

The Smart Shopper
Diabetes Cookbook

Strategies for Stress-Free Meals
from the Deli Counter, Freezer, Salad Bar, and Grocery Shelves

by ROBYN WEBB, MS

Director, Book Publishing, Abe Ogden; *Managing Editor,* Greg Guthrie; *Acquisitions Editor,* Victor Van Beuren; *Editor,* Rebekah Renshaw; *Production Manager,* Melissa Sprott; *Composition,* Circle Graphics; *Cover Design, Rachel Freedman at* SportCreative; *Photographer,* Renee Comet; Printer: RR Donnelly.

Printed in the United States of America
1 3 5 7 9 10 8 6 4 2

The suggestions and information contained in this publication are generally consistent with the *Clinical Practice Recommendations* and other policies of the American Diabetes Association, but they do not represent the policy or position of the Association or any of its boards or committees. Reasonable steps have been taken to ensure the accuracy of the information presented. However, the American Diabetes Association cannot ensure the safety or efficacy of any product or service described in this publication. Individuals are advised to consult a physician or other appropriate health care professional before undertaking any diet or exercise program or taking any medication referred to in this publication. Professionals must use and apply their own professional judgment, experience, and training and should not rely solely on the information contained in this publication before prescribing any diet, exercise, or medication. The American Diabetes Association—its officers, directors, employees, volunteers, and members—assumes no responsibility or liability for personal or other injury, loss, or damage that may result from the suggestions or information in this publication.

♾ The paper in this publication meets the requirements of the ANSI Standard Z39.48-1992 (permanence of paper).

ADA titles may be purchased for business or promotional use or for special sales. To purchase more than 50 copies of this book at a discount, or for custom editions of this book with your logo, contact the American Diabetes Association at the address below, at booksales@diabetes.org, or by calling 703-299-2046.

American Diabetes Association
1701 North Beauregard Street
Alexandria, Virginia 22311

DOI: 10.2337/9781580404945

Library of Congress Cataloging-in-Publication Data

Webb, Robin.
    / Robin Webb.
    pages cm
 Includes bibliographical references and index.
 ISBN 978-1-58040-494-5 (alk. paper)
 1. Diabetes--Diet therapy--Recipes. 2. Menus. I. Title.
 RC662.W353 2013
 641.5'6314--dc23
                        2012051163

TABLE OF CONTENTS

To my late mother Ruth, my truest,
best, and smartest grocery shopping partner.

ACKNOWLEDGMENTS

People say I make writing cookbooks look effortless. That's a grand compliment considering I've written so many. Truth be told, producing a cookbook is not for the fainthearted. You must have an extraordinary amount of support from team players. Without them, none of my books would have become realities.

The publishing world has changed a bit from when I first starting writing in the early 90's. But one thing that hasn't changed is the undying amount of support I have received for so many years from the American Diabetes Association. The dynamic team of Abe Ogden, Rebekah Renshaw, and Greg Guthrie has given me the ultimate platform from which to really make a difference in the lives of people with diabetes and their families. The guidance and wisdom has given me a partnership I hold very dear.

I think that while the text and recipes of a cookbook are of course critically important, first impressions really do count. And I hold my favorite food photographer and stylist on a pedestal as the best team to create that beautiful impression. Renee Comet and Lisa Cherkasky have tremendous talent and I know how fortunate I am to have them in my inner circle. Their relentless pursuit of perfection is a marvel to observe.

So many thanks to Circle Graphics, for the beautiful design and layout of the book. A cookbook is much more than just a bunch of recipes on a page and they have truly captured the essence of *The Smart Shopper Diabetes Cookbook*.

To my super agent, Beth Shepard, who is more than just an agent, but is really part of my family. I feel like I've "grown up" with her throughout the years as she steadfastly supports me through thick and thin and always has a clear vision as to what direction I should take. She leads me down the right path every time.

It's comforting when your team of recipe testers can't sit still until I write another book and we get going on the next project. Fortunately I keep them very busy. Led by the hardest working duo I know, Ramzi Faris and Cecilia Stoute, these two fine team leaders kept everyone working at a great pace and demanded only the most meticulous testing. I am truly indebted to them for helping me to coordinate this entire book.

Thank you to all the local supermarkets in the DC metro area. I enjoyed perusing your aisles, inspecting your salad bars, peering into your delis, and opening and closing all those freezer doors! You've come a long way—thank you for providing better and healthier selections with every passing year.

And finally to you dear reader, you've been at my side from my very first cookbook so many years ago. It is with you that I share my ultimate passion: creating sensational food for people with diabetes.

INTRODUCTION
Nutritional Information for this Book

There has never been a one-size-fits-all nutritional approach for people with diabetes. Thank goodness for that! This cookbook emphasizes the fabulous ways you can prepare your meals with less stress and more flavor. However, every single person is different, and so are his or her nutrition needs. The nutrient analysis for each recipe is in accordance with the American Diabetes Association guidelines, but you may have some additional questions about the ingredients used for the recipes. In this section I'll discuss some of the major concerns people with diabetes have.

In my book, every effort was made to highlight true convenience foods that you could replicate if you needed to prepare that food from scratch. That's the true test of whether a food is processed or not. For example, if you soaked and cooked your own beans, they would look similar (with some variance in texture) to the canned version. Purchasing already chopped carrots would look the same as if you cut them yourself. I kept true to developing recipes with wholesome ingredients that come in a form that's more convenient, especially helpful when you are very busy and short on time or skill.

Somewhere along the line carbohydrates became the bad guy. Yes, solid scientific research shows that carbohydrates do indeed affect blood sugar levels more than fat and proteins; however, a complete refusal to include a healthy level of carbohydrates can do more harm than good.

When looking over these recipes, you will see that some of them are higher in carbohydrates than others. If you look carefully, these recipes are also high in fiber. Fiber is critical to the management of blood sugar levels. Fiber also aids weight control and can promote a healthy digestive system, which is important for overall health. So, don't immediately discount high carbohydrate recipes. With a little help from your registered dietitian, most recipes can be worked into your already established meal plan quite nicely.

Many of the recipes in this book are main meal ideas. The vegetarian main dishes will certainly be higher in overall grams of carbohydrate. So for the recipes based in whole grains, pastas (whole grain pasta is recommended), and beans, they can be served in a smaller portion as a side dish rather than as a main meal to fit into your plan accordingly.

Because there are many approaches to regulating blood sugar levels, this book makes no attempt to exclude high fiber and nutrient-rich recipes that happen to be higher in grams of carbohydrates than some other recipes. I worked hard to make sure there would be enough recipes for everyone to enjoy.

The American Diabetes Association nutritional guidelines were developed to help people with diabetes make the best possible daily food choices. When it comes to saturated fat, ADA guidelines have a tight limit on the amount a recipe can contain, while still providing delicious flavor. Good quality olive oil and tasty olives, a small amount of nuts, fiber-rich avocados, and the use of lean cuts of animal protein in reasonable portions are the main sources of total fat grams. The only fat-free products I use are small amounts of sour cream, mayonnaise, and some cheeses. They are added to retain the familiarity one has with a texture of a dish. The fat-free products provided today are so much better in quality than in the past. Any solid fat may be a small amount of non-hydrogenated butter spread. This is used so I may adhere to ADA guidelines because other fat-containing ingredients in the same recipe are of more importance to the overall quality of the recipe and should not be changed from their original state.

I worked hard to balance the flavors of each recipe right alongside creating recipes appropriate for this book. When it comes to sodium, I worked in earnest to keep the grams down. I do add salt to many of the recipes as it truly does bring out the flavors of the dish. I prefer Kosher salt for most of my needs as it's inexpensive and the grains are cut a bit thicker so the salt can cover more ground. Feel free to eliminate it if you prefer. I've also worked in a few of my favorite salt-free blends that are truly tasty. So, whether I add salt or not depends on the nature of the recipe, but you can decide for yourself.

I hope you will use this book as an opportunity to widen your culinary horizons and include new ideas in your food plan. Rather than dismissing any recipe based on what you have heard or hasn't presently been part of your plan, I urge you to discuss all these matters with a registered dietitian. I want you to be successful in the management of your diabetes and it is my humble wish that this book be a part of that management.

Yours in health,

Robyn Webb

Healthful Cooking Suggestions

Use More Often . . .

More nonstarchy vegetables **WHY?** *Increases fiber, reduces carbohydrate and calories*	More whole grains (breads, pastas, brown rice) instead of refined (white) grains **WHY?** *Increases fiber and some vitamins and minerals*	More herbs and spices **WHY?** *Reduces sodium and increases flavors*	More fish and seafood **WHY?** *Reduces saturated fat and provides healthful fat*
Small amounts of oil (olive and other vegetable and nut oils) or no-trans-fat tub margarine to replace butter or margarine **WHY?** *Reduces saturated and trans fats*	Egg substitute or egg whites to replace part or all of the eggs **WHY?** *Reduces saturated fat*	Reduced-fat or fat-free salad dressings or vinaigrettes to replace regular salad dressings **WHY?** *Reduces saturated fat*	Low-fat or fat-free dairy products (milk, yogurt) instead of regular dairy products **WHY?** *Reduces saturated fat*
Fat-free cream cheese and fat-free sour cream to replace part or all of the regular or reduced-fat cream cheese and sour cream **WHY?** *Reduces saturated fat*	Reduced-sodium or low-sodium broths/stocks (or homemade with no added salt) instead of regular canned or boxed broths **WHY?** *Reduces sodium*	Fresh and unsalted vegetables and dried cooked beans. Drain and rinse canned items (use reduced-sodium or no-salt-added products when possible). **WHY?** *Reduces sodium*	

. . . and less often

Fewer regular or lower-fat hard (yellow) cheeses. Think of them as garnishes, not the main event. **WHY?** *Reduces saturated fat and sodium*	Fewer deli meats such as sliced ham, salami, and smoked turkey **WHY?** *Reduces sodium*	Less meat, especially regular ground and other higher-fat meat **WHY?** *Reduces saturated fat*	Less added salt. Taste the food before adding any at the stove or table. **WHY?** *Reduces sodium*

CHAPTER 1
A Walk through the Grocery Aisles & Labels

I have a good friend who dislikes grocery shopping. In fact, she loathes it. She says she spends way too much time in the store only to bring home a costly grocery receipt with no ability to actually make meals from her purchases. She feels overwhelmed and disorganized. And she's not alone. In all my years as a nutritionist and culinary instructor, I've met countless people who share my friend's hatred of grocery shopping.

There is an easier way to ease those feelings about the supermarket. *The Smart Shopper Diabetes Cookbook* can help you organize your shopping experience so it's more enjoyable and less of a dreaded task. With a well-stocked pantry that includes herbs and spices, oils and vinegars, and other basic condiments, all it takes is a smart system to create all of the recipes in this book. Think about other areas of your life where you have organizational success. Whether it's your finances, your clothes closet, or your personal papers, I'll bet you have some sort of system that makes it all work. The grocery shopping experience is no different and this book helps puts the business of building daily meals into a workable system.

Rather than wander aimlessly through the aisles of the market, try thinking of the supermarket as four zones: shelf stable, frozen foods, deli, and salad bar. Once you think of the grocery in a strategic way, your trips will become successful and much less stressful.

Sections on fabulous quick soups and delectable desserts use a little bit from each area to create recipes you'll use over and over again. Organized in this fashion, you will become very familiar with the products offered in each of these sections and familiarity will give you a higher level of comfort with the entire process of meal planning.

The shelf stable section of the book is the largest, on purpose. Once you can establish a really good pantry system, there is never an excuse not to put together a nutritious meal. How many times have you started to prepare a recipe and find out you are missing some of the basics like canned tomatoes or ground spices? This section of the book prepares you to plan meals that are ready without stopping at the store on the way home from work. Wouldn't it be a real time saver if you could peer into your pantry and make creative dishes from what's already in there?

The freezer section of the market is more than just ice cream and frozen waffles. Frozen vegetables are just as good, and in some cases, more nutritious than fresh. It's wise to stock up on them because vegetables should play a vital role in any meal. I've made use of other freezer staples, such as frozen fruit, shrimp, chicken, filo dough, and pastas. While you may have strived to only include fresh foods in your meal plan, don't overlook frozen versions.

I remember when salad bars first made their debut in the grocery store. Back then, we all thought this was a novelty. In today's busy world, while it's certainly great to chop, slice, and dice all your fresh vegetables and fruits, sometimes you just don't have the time. While some may argue purchasing already cut up vegetables and fruit is more expensive than doing it yourself, take another look. Think about the times you have purchased whole produce only to have it go bad because you weren't able to eat it before it spoiled.

What about cooking for one or two? The produce department hasn't exactly kept up with the single serving idea and often you had to contend with eating broccoli five times in a row just to finish the bunch. Today's salad bars often have canned beans, grains, shredded Parmesan cheese, and so much more. When you just need a small amount of something, it's a good idea to really put your local salad bar to use.

Think the deli section is just for sandwich fillings? Think again. Today's delis are a lot like today's salad bars; so much better than years before. I've created wonderful ways to use lower sodium lean meats and healthy prepared salads from your store's deli. Don't have time to roast a whole turkey or chicken? Check out what's available in the deli. The time you save will be well worth it. When you purchase only what you need, you will start to notice your savings add up.

To bring the theme of organization and a smart system full circle, this book is also a menu planner for people with diabetes. You'll learn how to pair my creations with suggestions to make a complete meal. Eating for your health has never been easier or tastier. With the menu planner you will be able to take the guidelines and suggestions of your health professional and incorporate those recommendations into your daily life.

It is my hope that this book lives in your kitchen, deservedly earning all those creases and stains of frequent use. It's my hope that the entire process of planning meals from making a list, to the grocery shopping and preparation becomes more second nature with a lot less effort. It is my hope that you will cook often to feed yourself and your family with the very best returns for good health and delicious meals.

FOOD LABELS

MANY FOOD LABELS IN THE GROCERY STORE use terms that can be confusing. To help you shop and eat better, here is a list of the common terms as defined by the Food and Drug Administration.

Sugar

Sugar Free: Less than 0.5 gram of sugar per serving.

No Added Sugar, Without Added Sugar, No Sugar Added: This does not mean the same as "sugar free." A label bearing these words means that no sugars were added during processing, or that processing does not increase the sugar content above the amount the ingredients naturally contain. Consult the nutrition information panel to see the total amount of sugar in this product.

Reduced Sugar: At least 25% less sugar per serving than the regular product.

Calories

Calorie Free: Fewer than 5 calories per serving.

Low Calorie: 40 calories or less per serving. (If servings are smaller than 30 grams, or smaller than 2 tablespoons, this means 40 calories or less per 50 grams of food.)

Reduced Calorie, Fewer Calories: At least 25% fewer calories per serving than the regular product.

Fat

Fat Free, Nonfat: Less than 0.5 gram of fat per serving.

Low Fat: 3 grams or less of fat per serving. (If servings are smaller than 30 grams, or smaller than 2 tablespoons, this means 3 grams or less of fat per 50 grams of food.)

Reduced Fat, Less Fat: At least 25% less fat per serving than the regular product.

Cholesterol

Cholesterol Free: Less than 2 milligrams of cholesterol, and 2 grams or less of saturated fat per serving.

Low Cholesterol: 20 milligrams or less of cholesterol, and 2 grams or less of saturated fat per serving.

Reduced Cholesterol, Less Cholesterol: At least 25% less cholesterol, and 2 grams or less of saturated fat per serving than the regular product.

Sodium

Sodium Free: Less than 5 milligrams of sodium per serving.

Low Sodium: 140 milligrams or less of sodium per serving.

Very Low Sodium: 35 milligrams or less of sodium per serving.

Reduced Sodium, Less Sodium: At least 25% less sodium per serving than the regular product.

Light or Lite Foods

Foods that are labeled "Light" or "Lite" are usually either lower in fat or lower in calories than the regular product. Some products may also be lower in sodium. Check the nutrition information label on the back of the product to make sure.

Meat and Poultry

Lean: Less than 10 grams of fat, 4.5 grams or less of saturated fat, and less than 95 milligrams of cholesterol per serving and per 100 grams.

Extra Lean: Less than 5 grams of fat, less than 2 grams of saturated fat, and less than 95 milligrams of cholesterol per serving and per 100 grams.

CHAPTER 2
Soups in a Snap

oups may be my favorite recipes in this book. Not to mention how easy they are to prepare. Much of the work happens on the stove during a simmering session. And by making use of all the sections of the market: deli, salad bar, shelf, and frozen, most of the laborious chopping, slicing, and dicing is gone.

Many of the soups here can be served as a main meal. I generously use a lot of beans and lentils in these recipes as they act as blank canvasses to showcase different flavors. For example, *Garlicky Chickpea Soup* (page 26) and *Indian Chickpea Stew* (page 27) make use of the wonderful garbanzo bean, but they veer off into two different flavor profiles. I did this purposely throughout this chapter to build a good "soup foundation" in which to work. All you need to do is get the basics: a bean, some vegetables, broth, and your choice of spices and herbs.

Other soups such as the *Tortilla Soup* (page 23) make good use of prepared rotisserie chicken, while *Italian Ravioli Soup* (page 24) is a clever use of frozen pasta. For those of you who enjoy a cool appetizer soup, I think you'll really savor *Ginger Honeydew Soup* (page 28), a real palate teaser!

Here are a few tips for making soup preparation even easier:

1. Prepare soups in a heavy-bottomed saucepan. As you sauté onions and garlic, you don't want them to burn, so a pot with a sturdy bottom is a must.

2. Make sure your pot is big enough for soups to simmer properly. Trying to cram vegetables, beans, lean protein, plus broth and canned tomatoes into a small pot

is frustrating and, ultimately, futile. I recommend a 3–4 quart pot for most of the recipes in this chapter.

3. For best results, even if you use pre-chopped vegetables from the salad bar, make sure your vegetables are close in size to one another. You want to avoid large chunks of onions in contrast to teeny pieces of carrot. You want to be able to taste all of the vegetables in one spoonful.

4. Soups will taste better if you let the onions cook the full amount of time called for in the recipe. If you sauté them too quickly, they won't develop that rich, caramelized base for your soup. You can combine garlic and onions together in a sauté, but never sauté garlic alone as it is prone to burning and tasting bitter.

5. Almost all these soups freeze well and I encourage you to do just that. You'll always be prepared with soup when the mood strikes you. For best results, don't freeze the full amount of soup in one container. Instead, section the soup into at least 3 portions using heavy, microwaveable, Ziploc bags to freeze them. Or freeze them in individual servings if that's more convenient.

6. Freeze the soups by stacking the Ziploc bags on each other and be sure to label and date them. Use frozen, homemade soups within 3–4 months for best results. You can reheat by defrosting the soup overnight in the refrigerator and then heat or microwave the soup in the Ziploc bag with the bag slightly opened.

WINTER CHICKPEA SOUP

Servings: 5   Serving Size: 1 cup   Prep Time: 10 minutes   Cook Time: 30 minutes

I'm into big bowls of satisfying soup that have all the ingredients I need for a meal. I'd pair this hearty soup with a green crisp salad and perhaps some warm unsweetened applesauce on the side!

2 teaspoons	olive oil
1/2 cup	chopped onion
1 tablespoon	chili powder
1 teaspoon	dry mustard
1 tablespoon	all-purpose flour
1 1/2 cups	low-fat, reduced-sodium chicken broth
1 tablespoon	molasses
1 tablespoon	red wine vinegar
1 (15-ounce) can	chickpeas, drained
1 (14.5-ounce) can	chopped tomatoes
1/4 teaspoon	Kosher salt
1/4 teaspoon	freshly ground black pepper
	juice from 1/2 lemon
1/3 cup	shredded Fontina cheese

1 Heat the oil in a large saucepan over medium heat. Add the onion and sauté for 3 minutes. Add in the chili powder and mustard and sauté for 1 minute. Add in the flour and sauté for 1 minute, coating the onion with the flour. Add in the chicken broth, molasses, and red wine vinegar. Bring to a boil. Lower the heat and simmer for 20 minutes.

2 Add in the chickpeas and tomatoes and simmer for 10 minutes. Season with salt and pepper. Squeeze in the fresh lemon juice. Top each bowl with Fontina cheese.

Exchanges/Choices

1 Starch	**Calories**	175	**Cholesterol**	10 mg	**Total Carbohydrate**	24 g	
1 Vegetable	Calories from Fat	55	**Sodium**	530 mg	Dietary Fiber	6 g	
1 Lean Meat	**Total Fat**	6.0 g	**Potassium**	475 mg	Sugars	8 g	
1/2 Fat	Saturated Fat	1.8 g			**Protein**	8 g	
	Trans Fat	0.0 g			**Phosphorus**	150 mg	

MAIN DISH BLACK BEAN SOUP

Servings: 9   Serving Size: 1 cup   Prep Time: 15 minutes   Cook Time: 15 minutes

When I want a hot soup in the winter, a steaming bowl of black bean soup hits the spot. By using practically everything you already have on your pantry shelves, you'll actually be glad when the temperature dips so you can prepare this oh-so-simple and satisfying cold weather dish.

2 teaspoons	olive oil
1 small	onion, chopped
1	garlic clove, minced
1 tablespoon	mild or hot chili powder
2 teaspoons	ground cumin
1/2 teaspoon	dried oregano
1/2 teaspoon	Kosher salt
1/4 teaspoon	freshly ground black pepper
3 (15-ounce) cans	no-salt-added black beans
1 cup	low-fat, reduced-sodium chicken broth
1/2 cup	dry red wine
1/4 cup	plain, non-fat yogurt
2 tablespoons	finely chopped red onion

1. Heat the oil in a large saucepan over medium heat. Add the onion and garlic and sauté for 4 minutes. Add the chili powder, cumin, oregano, salt, and pepper and sauté for 2 minutes.

2. Puree two of the cans of beans with their liquid. Drain and rinse the remaining can of beans. Add the pureed beans, whole beans, broth, and red wine to the saucepan and bring the soup to a simmer. Simmer on low heat for about 10 minutes.

3. Stir the yogurt until smooth. Ladle the soup into individual bowls. Garnish each bowl with a drizzle of yogurt and some chopped red onion.

Exchanges/Choices

1 1/2 Starch	**Calories**	140	**Cholesterol**	0 mg	**Total Carbohydrate**	23 g
1 Lean Meat	Calories from Fat	15	**Sodium**	190 mg	Dietary Fiber	7 g
	Total Fat	1.5 g	**Potassium**	420 mg	Sugars	3 g
	Saturated Fat	0.3 g			**Protein**	8 g
	Trans Fat	0.0 g			**Phosphorus**	170 mg

CANNELLINI BEAN SOUP

Servings: 7   Serving Size: 1 cup   Prep Time: 5 minutes   Cook Time: 20 minutes

When I first began to seriously cook, the only beans I was familiar with were baked beans! If you open my pantry today, it's jam packed with every kind of bean you can imagine. Among my very favorite bean is the cannellini. For many years, I used them solely in salads, but in recent years, I've started adding them to soups. They have a lovely appearance and great texture.

1 teaspoon	olive oil
1/2 cup	chopped onion
1	garlic clove, minced
2 cans (15-ounce)	no-salt-added cannellini beans
1 can (14.5-ounce)	diced tomatoes
2/3 cup	chopped low-sodium ham (cut from a 1/4-inch chunk from the deli, save any excess for another use)
1 can (14.5-ounce)	low-fat, reduced-sodium beef broth
1 cup	fresh spinach leaves, chopped (salad bar)
1	fresh lemon
1/4 teaspoon	Kosher or sea salt
1/4 teaspoon	freshly ground black pepper

1. Heat the oil in a saucepan over medium heat. Add the onion and garlic and sauté for 5 minutes. Puree one can of the cannellini beans with their liquid in a food processor or blender. Drain and rinse the other can of beans. Add the beans to the saucepan.

2. Add in the diced tomatoes, ham, beef broth, and spinach and bring to a boil. Reduce the heat and simmer on low for 10 minutes.

3. Squeeze the juice from the lemon and add to the saucepan. Season the soup with salt and pepper.

Exchanges/Choices

1 Starch	**Calories**	145	**Cholesterol**	5 mg	**Total Carbohydrate**	22 g
1 Vegetable	Calories from Fat	20	**Sodium**	410 mg	Dietary Fiber	6 g
1 Lean Meat	**Total Fat**	2.0 g	**Potassium**	505 mg	Sugars	4 g
	Saturated Fat	0.4 g			**Protein**	10 g
	Trans Fat	0.0 g			**Phosphorus**	170 mg

REFRIED BEAN SOUP

Servings: 6 | Serving Size: 1 cup | Prep Time: 15 minutes | Cook Time: 20 minutes

Refried beans are so delicious; however, traditional refried beans are loaded with fat and aren't a choice for healthy cooking. I remember when fat-free canned refried beans made their appearance on store shelves several years ago. It was with trepidation that I opened my first can expecting something mediocre. To my surprise, the beans were good! Here they are added to a cumin- and oregano-spiked soup topped with a touch of extra sharp cheese and fresh chopped tomatoes.

1 tablespoon	olive oil
2 cups	chopped onion
3	garlic cloves, minced
1 teaspoon	ground cumin
1 teaspoon	dried oregano
1/4 teaspoon	freshly ground black pepper
3 cups	low-fat, low-sodium chicken broth
1 (16-ounce) can plus 3/4 cup	fat-free refried beans
1/2 cup	shredded extra sharp reduced-fat cheddar cheese (such as Cabot 50% reduced)
1/2 cup	finely minced tomato

1. Heat the oil in a large saucepan over medium heat. Add the onion and garlic and sauté for 4 minutes. Add the cumin, oregano, and pepper and sauté for 1 minute.

2. Add in the broth and beans and mix well. Simmer on low heat for about 10 minutes.

3. Ladle into individual bowls and top with cheddar cheese and minced tomato.

Exchanges/Choices

1 Starch	**Calories**	165	**Cholesterol**	5 mg	**Total Carbohydrate**	21 g
1 Vegetable	Calories from Fat	40	**Sodium**	570 mg	Dietary Fiber	6 g
1 Lean Meat	**Total Fat**	4.5 g	**Potassium**	600 mg	Sugars	4 g
1/2 Fat	Saturated Fat	1.5 g			**Protein**	10 g
	Trans Fat	0.0 g			**Phosphorus**	205 mg

PUMPKIN SOUP

Servings: 5 | **Serving Size:** 1 cup | **Prep Time:** 5 minutes | **Cook Time:** 15 minutes

Pumpkin is the only vegetable I refuse to cook. I detest messing with fresh pumpkin unless I'm carving it for the front porch at Halloween. Fortunately, canned pumpkin is a cook's dream. With the same nutritional profile as fresh, I keep canned pumpkin on my shelf year round.

2 teaspoons	olive oil
1/2 cup	diced onion
1	garlic clove, minced
1 (16-ounce) can	solid, packed pumpkin (**not** pumpkin pie filling)
1 1/2 cups	low-fat, reduced-sodium chicken broth
1 cup	fat-free evaporated milk
1/4 teaspoon	Kosher or sea salt
1/8 teaspoon	freshly ground black pepper
1/4 cup	grated fresh Parmesan cheese
2 tablespoons	chopped toasted pistachios or almonds

1. Heat the oil in a large saucepan over medium heat. Add the onion and garlic and sauté for 3 minutes.

2. Add in the pumpkin and broth and cook for about 5 minutes. Add in the milk and simmer on low heat for 3 minutes. Add in the salt, pepper, and Parmesan cheese and heat for 1 minute.

3. Ladle into individual bowls and top with pistachios or almonds.

Exchanges/Choices

1/2 Starch
1/2 Fat-Free Milk
1/2 Fat

Calories	125	**Cholesterol**	5 mg	**Total Carbohydrate**	16 g
Calories from Fat	35	**Sodium**	345 mg	Dietary Fiber	3 g
Total Fat	4.0 g	**Potassium**	465 mg	Sugars	10 g
Saturated Fat	1.0 g			**Protein**	7 g
Trans Fat	0.0 g			**Phosphorus**	175 mg

CHICKPEA TOMATO SOUP

Servings: 10   Serving Size: 1 cup   Prep Time: 8 minutes   Cook Time: 50 minutes

Shelf-stable low-sodium vegetable juice is more than just a beverage. Here, I've combined the juice with other shelf-stable ingredients for this warm and inviting soup. My secret weapon is a commercially prepared pesto that gives the soup an extra lift.

1 tablespoon	olive oil
1 large	onion, diced
2	garlic cloves, minced
1 medium	red pepper, cored, seeded, and diced
3 cups	low-fat, reduced-sodium chicken broth
1 1/2 cups	low-sodium vegetable juice
1 (28-ounce) can	whole plum tomatoes
1 (15-ounce) can	chickpeas, drained and rinsed
1/4 cup	prepared pesto
1/4 teaspoon	freshly ground black pepper
1/8 teaspoon	crushed red pepper flakes
1 tablespoon	fresh lemon juice

1. Heat the olive oil in a large saucepot over medium-high heat. Add in the onion and sauté on medium-low heat for about 10 minutes. Add the garlic and red pepper and sauté for 3 minutes.

2. Add in the broth and vegetable juice and bring to a boil. Meanwhile, add the canned tomatoes with their juice to a large bowl. With your hands, crush the tomatoes into small pieces. Add the tomatoes to the pot and lower the heat to simmer. Simmer the soup for 20 minutes.

3. Add in the chickpeas and cook for another 5 minutes. Stir in the pesto, pepper, and crushed red pepper. Remove the soup from the heat and add the lemon juice.

Exchanges/Choices

1/2 Starch	**Calories**	115	**Cholesterol**	0 mg	**Total Carbohydrate**	16 g
2 Vegetable	Calories from Fat	35	**Sodium**	480 mg	Dietary Fiber	4 g
1/2 Fat	**Total Fat**	4.0 g	**Potassium**	420 mg	Sugars	6 g
	Saturated Fat	0.6 g			**Protein**	5 g
	Trans Fat	0.0 g			**Phosphorus**	100 mg

MIXED MUSHROOM SOUP

Servings: 12   Serving Size: 1 cup   Prep Time: 15 minutes   Cook Time: 1 hour

One of the best things about mushrooms is all the wonderful varieties they come in. And the use of both fresh and dried mushrooms in the same recipe provides an instant depth of flavor. What I love about using dried mushrooms is that they last a very long time on your pantry shelf and are so easy to use. The elegant taste of white wine lingers beautifully on your palate making it perfect for entertaining your guests.

1 cup	very hot water
1 (2-ounce) package	dried porcini mushrooms
1 1/2 tablespoons	olive oil
2 large	onions, chopped
6	garlic cloves, minced
7 cups	sliced mushrooms (from salad bar or produce section)
1 cup	dry white wine
4 cups	low-fat, reduced-sodium chicken broth
1 cup	water
1 medium	russet potato, peeled and cubed
1/2 teaspoon	kosher salt
1/4 teaspoon	freshly ground black pepper

Garnish

1/4 cup	minced chives
1/4 cup	crème fraiche or 1/2 cup plain, non-fat yogurt

1. In a heatproof bowl, pour the hot water over the porcini mushrooms and set aside for 15 minutes.

2. Heat the olive oil in a 6-quart saucepan over medium heat. Add the onions and sauté for 6–7 minutes. Add the garlic and sauté for 3 minutes until fragrant. Add in the fresh mushrooms and sauté for 5–6 minutes. Add in the wine and cook until wine has reduced in volume by one half, about 10 minutes.

3. Add in the broth, water, potatoes, and porcini mushrooms with their water and bring to a boil. Reduce the heat and simmer for 30 minutes.

4. Puree the soup in batches in the food processor or blender. Return the soup to the saucepan. Season with salt and pepper. Top with chives and swirl 1 teaspoon of crème fraiche or yogurt into each bowl of soup.

Exchanges/Choices

2 Vegetable	**Calories**	90	**Cholesterol**	5 mg	**Total Carbohydrate**	12 g
1 Fat	Calories from Fat	30	**Sodium**	255 mg	Dietary Fiber	2 g
	Total Fat	3.5 g	**Potassium**	365 mg	Sugars	3 g
	Saturated Fat	1.4 g			**Protein**	3 g
	Trans Fat	0.0 g			**Phosphorus**	80 mg

CHICKPEAS WITH GREENS SOUP

Servings: 8   Serving Size: 1 cup   Prep Time: 20 minutes   Cook Time: 30 minutes

My favorite soups are of Italian origin. Here I go beyond the familiar soups like Minestrone, to present one of the homiest of the country's soups: chickpeas and greens. It's so simple when you stop off at the salad bar for prewashed spinach and already sliced carrots. Toss in a few cans of chickpeas and a few shelf-stable dried spices and you'll be transported to Italy in no time.

1 tablespoon	olive oil
1 large	onion, diced
2	garlic cloves, minced
1 cup	sliced carrots (salad bar)
1/2 teaspoon	dried thyme
1/2 teaspoon	dried basil
	pinch crushed red pepper flakes
2 (15-ounce) cans	chickpeas, drained and rinsed
4 cups	low-fat, reduced-sodium chicken broth
4 cups	torn spinach (salad bar)
	juice from 1/2 lemon
1/2 teaspoon	Kosher salt
1/4 teaspoon	freshly ground black pepper

1. Heat the oil in a large saucepot over medium heat. Add the onion and garlic and sauté for 6–7 minutes. Add in the carrots and sauté for 5 minutes. Add in the thyme, basil, and crushed red pepper and sauté for 1 minute.

2. Add in the chickpeas and broth and bring to a boil. Lower the heat and simmer for 15 minutes. Puree half the soup in a food processor or blender. Return the pureed mixture to the soup. Add in the greens and cook for 1–2 minutes until wilted. Add in the lemon juice, salt, and pepper and remove from the heat.

Exchanges/Choices

1 Starch	**Calories**	145	**Cholesterol**	0 mg	**Total Carbohydrate**	23 g
1 Vegetable	Calories from Fat	30	**Sodium**	505 mg	Dietary Fiber	6 g
1 Lean Meat	**Total Fat**	3.5 g	**Potassium**	445 mg	Sugars	6 g
	Saturated Fat	0.4 g			**Protein**	8 g
	Trans Fat	0.0 g			**Phosphorus**	140 mg

TOFU VEGETABLE SOUP

Servings: 9   Serving Size: 1 cup   Prep Time: 15 minutes   Cook Time: 15 minutes

Hate chopping cabbage? Well I do, and so I love it when the salad bar has fresh, shredded cabbage available. I almost prefer cooked cabbage to raw and this works so well in this soup redolent with fresh ginger. The finishing sauce of rice vinegar, soy sauce, and hot chili oil really gives this soup a punch.

1 pound	extra firm tofu, cut into 1/2-inch cubes (salad bar or packaged, drained)
1 tablespoon	cornstarch
1 tablespoon	sesame oil
1/2 cup	diced onion
2	garlic cloves, minced
1 tablespoon	grated ginger
1 cup	sliced carrot (salad bar)
3 cups	shredded cabbage (salad bar or produce section)
3 cups	low-fat, reduced-sodium chicken broth
2 tablespoons	rice vinegar
1 tablespoon	lite soy sauce
1/4 teaspoon	hot chili oil

1. Add the tofu to a large bowl. Sprinkle the tofu with the cornstarch and gently toss. Heat the sesame oil in a large Dutch oven over medium-high heat. Add the tofu and sauté on all sides for about 3–4 minutes or until lightly browned. With a slotted spoon remove the tofu to a plate and set aside. Reduce the heat to medium; add the onion and garlic and sauté for 3–4 minutes. Add the ginger and sauté for 2 minutes.

2. Add in the carrot, cabbage, and broth and bring to a boil. Lower the heat and simmer for 10 minutes. Add in the sautéed tofu, rice vinegar, soy sauce, and hot chili oil and simmer for 3 minutes.

Exchanges/Choices

1 Vegetable	**Calories**	90	**Cholesterol**	0 mg	**Total Carbohydrate**	7 g	
1 Med-Fat Meat	Calories from Fat	40	**Sodium**	260 mg	Dietary Fiber	2 g	
	Total Fat	4.5 g	**Potassium**	225 mg	Sugars	2 g	
	Saturated Fat	0.6 g			**Protein**	7 g	
	Trans Fat	0.0 g			**Phosphorus**	95 mg	

RED LENTIL SOUP

Servings: 4	Serving Size: 1 cup	Prep Time: 10 minutes	Cook Time: 25 minutes

A creamy and comforting soup. I think red lentils should always occupy your pantry shelf. Prettier than the usual brown or green lentils, this soup has not only great eye appeal, but the aroma of the ginger and the spices make this soup shine.

1 tablespoon	olive oil
1 small	onion, diced
2	garlic cloves, minced
1 small	red pepper, cored, seeded, and diced
1 teaspoon	grated fresh ginger
1 teaspoon	ground cumin
1/2 teaspoon	ground coriander
1/4 teaspoon	Kosher salt
1/4 teaspoon	cayenne pepper
1 cup	red lentils
2 1/2 cups	low-fat, reduced-sodium chicken broth
1/2 cup	fat-free evaporated milk

Garnish

1/4 cup	stirred fat-free plain yogurt
	ground cumin

1 Heat the oil in a saucepan over medium heat. Add the onion, garlic, and red pepper and sauté for 5 minutes. Add in the ginger, cumin, coriander, salt, and cayenne pepper and sauté for 2 minutes. Add in the lentils and stir to coat the lentils with the onions and seasonings.

2 Add in the broth and bring to a boil. Lower the heat to medium low and simmer until lentils are tender. Add the lentils and evaporated milk to a food processor or blender and blend until smooth. Return the soup to the saucepan and taste and correct the seasonings. Top each bowl with a swirl of yogurt and light dusting of cumin.

Exchanges/Choices

2 Starch
2 Lean Meat

Calories	245	**Cholesterol**	0 mg	**Total Carbohydrate**	36 g
Calories from Fat	35	**Sodium**	490 mg	Dietary Fiber	11 g
Total Fat	4.0 g	**Potassium**	805 mg	Sugars	10 g
Saturated Fat	0.6 g			**Protein**	17 g
Trans Fat	0.0 g			**Phosphorus**	340 mg

LENTIL AND POTATO STEW

Servings: 6   **Serving Size:** 1 cup   **Prep Time:** 10 minutes   **Cook Time:** 1 hour and 10 minutes

Lentils are about the easiest dry bean to cook, so be sure to include them on your pantry essential list. Everything in this soup should be on your must-have pantry list, so this hearty meal is ready whenever you are.

1 tablespoon	olive oil
1 medium	onion, chopped
4	garlic cloves, minced
1 teaspoon	dried basil
3/4 cup	lentils
2 cups	low-fat, reduced-sodium chicken broth
2 cups	water
1 cup	canned no-salt-added chopped tomatoes, undrained
3	jarred roasted yellow peppers, diced
1/2 teaspoon	Kosher salt
1/4 teaspoon	freshly ground black pepper
1/2 pound	red potatoes cut into 1/2-inch chunks

Garnish

1/2 cup	minced parsley
1/2 cup	plain non-fat yogurt

1. Heat the olive oil in a large saucepot over medium heat. Add the onion and garlic and sauté for 6–7 minutes. Add in the basil and lentils and sauté for 1 minute.

2. Add in the broth, water, tomatoes, roasted peppers, salt, and pepper. Bring to a boil over high heat, reduce the heat to simmer, and cook for about 20 minutes until lentils are just barely tender.

3. Add in the potatoes and cook over medium-low heat for 45 minutes until potatoes are tender. Taste and correct seasonings. Sprinkle with parsley and a spoonful of yogurt.

Exchanges/Choices

1 1/2 Starch	**Calories**	175	**Cholesterol**	0 mg	**Total Carbohydrate**	31 g
1 Vegetable	Calories from Fat	25	**Sodium**	395 mg	Dietary Fiber	7 g
1 Lean Meat	**Total Fat**	3.0 g	**Potassium**	690 mg	Sugars	7 g
	Saturated Fat	0.4 g			**Protein**	10 g
	Trans Fat	0.0 g			**Phosphorus**	215 mg

CREAMY BROCCOLI SOUP

Servings: 5   Serving Size: 1 cup   Prep Time: 10 minutes   Cook Time: 20 minutes

I've always loved cream soups, but they don't love my waistline! But by cleverly using a small amount of half and half, this soup is as creamy as its heavy counterpart. Frozen broccoli is perfect for this soup as it cooks up well and makes a nice puree.

2 teaspoons	olive oil
1 1/2 teaspoons	butter
1 medium	onion, chopped
3	garlic cloves, minced
2 tablespoons	all-purpose flour
1 teaspoon	dried thyme
1/4 teaspoon	dried oregano
	pinch crushed red pepper flakes
1 (10-ounce) package	frozen broccoli
1 1/2 cups	low-fat, reduced-sodium chicken broth
3/4 cup	1% milk
1/4 cup	half and half
2 teaspoons	grated fresh lemon zest
1/2 teaspoon	Kosher salt
1/4 teaspoon	freshly ground black pepper

Garnish

1/4 cup	chopped toasted hazelnuts

1. Heat the olive oil and butter in a large saucepan over medium heat. Add the onion and garlic and sauté for 6–7 minutes. Add in the flour, thyme, oregano, and crushed red pepper flakes and sauté until flour is incorporated into the onion mixture.

2. Add in the broccoli and broth and bring to a boil. Lower the heat and simmer for 10 minutes.

3. Add the broccoli mixture to a food processor or blender and add the milk. Puree until smooth.

4. Add the soup back to the saucepan and simmer over low heat for 3 minutes. Add in the half and half and lemon zest and simmer for 1 minute. Season with salt and pepper. Garnish with the hazelnuts.

Exchanges/Choices

1/2 Carbohydrate	**Calories**	140	**Cholesterol**	10 mg	**Total Carbohydrate**	12 g
1 Vegetable	Calories from Fat	70	**Sodium**	390 mg	Dietary Fiber	3 g
2 Fat	**Total Fat**	8.0 g	**Potassium**	310 mg	Sugars	4 g
	Saturated Fat	2.4 g			**Protein**	6 g
	Trans Fat	0.1 g			**Phosphorus**	115 mg

FALL BUTTERNUT SQUASH SOUP

As much as I love cooking fresh butternut squash, I have to honestly say how much I appreciate the convenient frozen butternut squash puree! No seeds or skin to remove. This creamy cumin-touched soup makes a great beginning to a special holiday meal.

1 tablespoon	olive oil
1 cup	diced onion
3	garlic cloves, minced
1 tablespoon	curry powder
1 tablespoon	brown sugar
1/2 teaspoon	ground cumin
1/8 teaspoon	cayenne pepper
3 (10-ounce) packages	frozen butternut squash puree, slightly thawed
4 cups	low-fat, reduced-sodium chicken broth
1/4 cup	half and half
1/2 teaspoon	Kosher salt
1/4 teaspoon	freshly ground black pepper

Garnish

1/4 cup	toasted chopped pistachio nuts

1. Heat the oil in a saucepot over medium heat. Add the onion and garlic and sauté for 6–7 minutes. Add in the curry powder, brown sugar, cumin, and cayenne pepper and sauté for 1 minute.

2. Add in the squash puree and broth and bring to a boil. Lower the heat and simmer for 10 minutes. Add in the half and half, salt, and pepper. Garnish with pistachio nuts.

Exchanges/Choices

1 Starch	**Calories**	130	**Cholesterol**	5 mg	**Total Carbohydrate**	19 g	
1 Vegetable	Calories from Fat	45	**Sodium**	440 mg	Dietary Fiber	3 g	
1 Fat	**Total Fat**	5.0 g	**Potassium**	370 mg	Sugars	6 g	
	Saturated Fat	1.2 g			**Protein**	3 g	
	Trans Fat	0.0 g			**Phosphorus**	75 mg	

LENTIL AND BROWN RICE STEW

Servings: 5   Serving Size: 1 cup   Prep Time: 15 minutes   Cook Time: 55 minutes

Look over these ingredients and I'm sure you have everything to make this hearty stew right now. A vegetarian's delight, shelf-stable broth, tomatoes, and an array of dry spices create this warm inviting winter stew that freezes great.

1 tablespoon	olive oil
1 large	onion, chopped
2	garlic cloves, minced
1 cup	chopped carrots (salad bar)
1 teaspoon	dried oregano
1 teaspoon	dried basil
1 cup	dried lentils
5 cups	fat-free, low-sodium chicken broth
1 (28-ounce) can	whole plum tomatoes, undrained
1 cup	frozen, cooked brown rice
1/4 teaspoon	freshly ground black pepper
1/4 teaspoon	crushed red pepper flakes

1. Heat the oil in a large saucepan over medium heat. Sauté the onions and garlic for about 5–6 minutes. Add in the carrots and sauté for 4 minutes.

2. Add in the oregano, basil, and lentils and sauté for 2 minutes. Add in the broth and bring to a boil.

3. Add the tomatoes to a large bowl. With your hands, crush the tomatoes into small pieces. Add the tomatoes and their juices to the saucepan. Lower the heat and simmer for 25 minutes, stirring occasionally. Add in the rice, pepper, and crushed red pepper flakes and simmer for 5–7 minutes.

Exchanges/Choices

2 Starch	**Calories**	260	**Cholesterol**	5 mg	**Total Carbohydrate**	45 g
2 Vegetable	Calories from Fat	35	**Sodium**	570 mg	Dietary Fiber	12 g
1 Lean Meat	**Total Fat**	4.0 g	**Potassium**	1035 mg	Sugars	9 g
	Saturated Fat	0.8 g			**Protein**	15 g
	Trans Fat	0.0 g			**Phosphorus**	285 mg

TORTILLA SOUP

Look around your kitchen right now, and I'll bet you have most all the ingredients for this delightfully spiced soup. All you need to do is pick up a roasted chicken and dinner is served!

1 tablespoon	olive oil
1 small	onion, diced
3	garlic cloves, minced
1 1/2 cups	shredded cooked chicken (from a rotisserie chicken, boned and skinned)
1 tablespoon	mild or hot chili powder
2 teaspoons	ground cumin
1/4 teaspoon	Kosher salt
1/4 teaspoon	freshly ground black pepper
4 cups	low-fat, low-sodium chicken broth
1 (14.5-ounce) can	diced tomatoes with chilies
1/2 cup	lightly crushed fat-free tortilla chips
1/4 cup	reduced-fat shredded Monterey Jack cheese

Garnish

	lime wedges

1. Heat the oil in a large saucepan over medium heat. Add the onion and garlic and sauté for 4 minutes. Add in the chicken, chili powder, ground cumin, salt, and pepper. Sauté for 3–4 minutes.

2. Add in the broth and tomatoes and bring to a boil. Reduce the heat and simmer for 15 minutes.

3. Ladle the soup into individual bowls and top with tortilla chips and cheese. Serve with lime wedges.

Exchanges/Choices

1/2 Starch	**Calories**	160	**Cholesterol**	45 mg	**Total Carbohydrate**	13 g
1 Vegetable	Calories from Fat	55	**Sodium**	575 mg	Dietary Fiber	2 g
2 Lean Meat	**Total Fat**	6.0 g	**Potassium**	390 mg	Sugars	4 g
1/2 Fat	Saturated Fat	1.7 g			**Protein**	15 g
	Trans Fat	0.0 g			**Phosphorus**	170 mg

ITALIAN RAVIOLI SOUP

Servings: 6　　Serving Size: 1 cup　　Prep Time: 20 minutes　　Cook Time: 25 minutes

When I was growing up, the neighbor next door would labor over making the most perfect ravioli every Sunday. She'd invite me over to watch and while it was intriguing, I never had a desire to work quite as hard as she did! Today, frozen ravioli is delicious without putting in all that effort. Here the ravioli gently float amidst fresh vegetables and shelf-stable tomatoes and broth with a touch of zesty Italian spices.

1 (9-oz) package	reduced-fat frozen ravioli (such as Buitoni)
1 tablespoon	olive oil
1 medium	onion, chopped
2	garlic cloves, minced
1/2 cup	diced red bell pepper
1/4 cup	diced celery
1 teaspoon	dried salt-free Italian seasoning
1 cup	shredded green cabbage
1 (15-ounce) can	diced canned Italian-style tomatoes, undrained
3 1/2 cups	low-fat, reduced-sodium chicken broth
1/2 cup	water
2 tablespoons	grated fresh Parmesan cheese

1. Boil the ravioli according to package directions. Drain and set aside.

2. Heat the oil in a large saucepot. Add the onion and sauté for 5–6 minutes. Add the garlic, red pepper, and celery and sauté for 3 minutes. Add in the Italian seasoning and sauté for 1 minute.

3. Add in the cabbage, canned tomatoes, broth, and water and bring to a boil. Lower the heat and simmer for 15 minutes. Add in the ravioli and simmer for 5 minutes. Sprinkle with Parmesan cheese.

Exchanges/Choices

1 Starch	**Calories**	180	**Cholesterol**	15 mg	**Total Carbohydrate**	26 g
2 Vegetable	Calories from Fat	45	**Sodium**	585 mg	Dietary Fiber	3 g
1 Fat	**Total Fat**	5.0 g	**Potassium**	360 mg	Sugars	6 g
	Saturated Fat	2.0 g			**Protein**	9 g
	Trans Fat	0.0 g			**Phosphorus**	105 mg

WHITE BEAN AND TURKEY SOUP

Servings: 6   Serving Size: 1 cup   Prep Time: 20 minutes   Cook Time: 45 minutes

Broaden your thinking when you purchase low-sodium deli turkey. Instead of a sandwich, toss turkey cubes into this comforting white bean soup. Ask for 2/3 pound of deli turkey cut in one chunk; when you get home, cut the turkey into 1/2-inch cubes. Any canned bean of your choice will work here, so try this with black, kidney, garbanzo, navy, or pinto beans.

1 tablespoon	olive oil
1 medium	onion, chopped
1 cup	diced carrots
2/3 cup	chopped celery
1/4 teaspoon	freshly ground black pepper
1/4 teaspoon	crushed red pepper flakes
3 1/2 cups	fat-free, low-sodium chicken broth
2 (15-ounce) cans	cannellini beans
2/3 pound	cooked low-sodium deli turkey, cut into 1/2-inch cubes
1 teaspoon	fresh minced thyme

1. Heat the oil in a large saucepot over medium-high heat. Add the onion and sauté for 5–6 minutes. Add the carrots, celery, pepper, and crushed red pepper and sauté for 3–4 minutes.

2. Add in the broth and bring to a boil. Lower the heat and simmer for 5 minutes.

3. Meanwhile, puree one can of the white beans with its liquid in a blender or food processor. Add to the soup and simmer for 10 minutes.

4. Drain and rinse the remaining can of beans. Add the drained beans, turkey, and thyme to the soup and simmer for 15 minutes.

Exchanges/Choices

1 Starch	**Calories**	205	**Cholesterol**	25 mg	**Total Carbohydrate**	24 g
1 Vegetable	Calories from Fat	30	**Sodium**	535 mg	Dietary Fiber	7 g
2 Lean Meat	**Total Fat**	3.5 g	**Potassium**	745 mg	Sugars	3 g
	Saturated Fat	0.7 g			**Protein**	19 g
	Trans Fat	0.0 g			**Phosphorus**	280 mg

GARLICKY CHICKPEA SOUP

Servings: 9   Serving Size: 1 cup   Prep Time: 20 minutes   Cook Time: 35 minutes

Garlic lovers rejoice! With everything that is shelf stable, just add a boatload of garlic and an onion and you have a main dish. To slip the skins off that many garlic cloves, add the cloves, unpeeled to a pot of boiling water. Turn the heat off and let the garlic stand in the water for 1 minute. Drain. The garlic skins will slip right off!

1 tablespoon	olive oil
1 large	onion, chopped
8	garlic cloves, minced
4 cups	low-fat, reduced-sodium chicken broth
1 teaspoon	dried crumbled rosemary
1/4 teaspoon	Kosher salt
1/4 teaspoon	freshly ground black pepper
1/4 teaspoon	crushed red pepper flakes
3 (15-ounce) cans	chickpeas, drained and rinsed
1 (14.5-ounce) can	diced tomatoes, undrained
1 tablespoon	good-quality balsamic vinegar

1. Heat the oil in a large saucepot over medium heat. Add the onions and garlic and sauté for about 10 minutes. Add in the remaining ingredients except the balsamic vinegar. Bring to a boil. Reduce the heat and simmer for 20 minutes.

2. Ladle about 3 cups of the soup into a food processor or blender. Puree the soup until smooth. Add back to the remaining soup in the pot. Add in the vinegar and simmer for 3 minutes.

Exchanges/Choices

1 1/2 Starch	**Calories**	180	**Cholesterol**	0	**Total Carbohydrate**	29 g
1 Vegetable	Calories from Fat	35	mg **Sodium**	490 mg	Dietary Fiber	7 g
1 Lean Meat	**Total Fat**	4.0 g	**Potassium**	450 mg	Sugars	7 g
	Saturated Fat	0.5 g			**Protein**	9 g
	Trans Fat	0.0 g			**Phosphorus**	175 mg

INDIAN CHICKPEA STEW

Although Italian cuisine does a fine job with chickpeas, I actually think Indian cuisine does it even better. Garam masala is a blend of many Indian spices and is available now at many major supermarkets in the spice section. With its five heady spices, chickpeas absorb a heavenly scent and flavor.

1 tablespoon	olive oil
1 medium	onion, chopped
2	garlic cloves, minced
1 teaspoon	sugar
1 teaspoon	curry powder
1/2 teaspoon	ground cumin
1/4 teaspoon	ground coriander
1/4 teaspoon	ground turmeric
1/8 teaspoon	ground cayenne pepper
2 (15-ounce) cans	diced tomatoes, drained
2 (15-ounce) cans	chickpeas, drained
1/2 teaspoon	Garam masala
1/4 teaspoon	Kosher salt
1/4 teaspoon	ground black pepper

1. Heat the oil in a large saucepan over medium heat. Add the onion and sauté for 7–8 minutes. Add the garlic and sauté for 2 minutes. Add in the sugar, curry powder, cumin, coriander, turmeric, and cayenne pepper. Sauté for 1 minute.

2. Add in the tomatoes and cook for 5 minutes. Add in the chickpeas, Garam masala, salt, and pepper. Simmer for 5 minutes.

Exchanges/Choices

2 Starch	**Calories**	280	**Cholesterol**	0 mg	**Total Carbohydrate**	45 g
2 Vegetable	Calories from Fat	65	**Sodium**	515 mg	Dietary Fiber	12 g
1 Lean Meat	**Total Fat**	7.0 g	**Potassium**	675 mg	Sugars	12 g
1/2 Fat	Saturated Fat	0.9 g			**Protein**	13 g
	Trans Fat	0.0 g			**Phosphorus**	250 mg

GINGER HONEYDEW SOUP

Cold soups are a wonderful way to begin a light meal. This emerald colored soup pairs nicely with a grain or pasta salad. The enticing ginger flavor will set your taste buds on fire for the next course.

2 1/2 cups	honeydew melon chunks (from the salad bar or fresh-cut melon)
2 tablespoons	pure maple syrup
2 tablespoons	fresh lemon juice
1 1/2 teaspoons	peeled, grated fresh ginger

Topping

1/3 cup	plain non-fat yogurt
2 teaspoons	finely minced crystallized ginger

1. Puree the honeydew melon, maple syrup, lemon juice, and fresh ginger in a blender or food processor until smooth. Pour into a bowl, cover, and refrigerate 1 hour.

2. For each serving, swirl in some yogurt and sprinkle with crystallized ginger.

Exchanges/Choices

1/2 Fruit
1 Carbohydrate

Calories	80	**Cholesterol**	0 mg	**Total Carbohydrate** 20 g
Calories from Fat	0	**Sodium**	35 mg	Dietary Fiber 1 g
Total Fat	0.0 g	**Potassium**	320 mg	Sugars 18 g
Saturated Fat	0.1 g			**Protein** 2 g
Trans Fat	0.0 g			**Phosphorus** 45 mg

COCONUT SOUP WITH SHRIMP AND SPINACH

Servings: 8   Serving Size: 1 cup   Prep Time: 5 minutes   Cook Time: 30 minutes

Although I love fresh spinach, I stock up on frozen spinach more than any other vegetable. Its versatility is endless and it looks beautiful floating in this soup enveloped in a creamy coconut milk and a spark of red curry paste.

2 teaspoons	vegetable oil
8 ounces	frozen red pepper and onion medley
2	garlic cloves, minced
2 teaspoons	red curry paste
2 (14-ounce) cans	fat-free, low-sodium chicken broth
1 cup	light coconut milk
2 teaspoons	brown sugar
2 teaspoons	fish sauce
1 pound	frozen medium uncooked shrimp, thawed and patted dry
1 (10-ounce) package	frozen leaf spinach, thawed and drained well
1/4 cup	sliced fresh Thai basil (optional)

1. Heat the oil in a large saucepan over medium heat. Add in the red pepper and onion medley and garlic and stir-fry for 3 minutes. Add in the curry paste and cook for 1 minute.

2. Stir in the broth, coconut milk, brown sugar, and fish sauce and bring to a boil. Reduce the heat and simmer, uncovered, for 20 minutes.

3. Add in the shrimp and spinach and cook for about 4 minutes until the shrimp are cooked through. Garnish each individual bowl of soup with Thai basil, if desired.

Exchanges/Choices

1 Vegetable 1 Lean Meat 1/2 Fat						
	Calories	105	**Cholesterol**	80 mg	**Total Carbohydrate**	7 g
	Calories from Fat	35	**Sodium**	575 mg	Dietary Fiber	1 g
	Total Fat	4.0 g	**Potassium**	330 mg	Sugars	3 g
	Saturated Fat	1.9 g			**Protein**	11 g
	Trans Fat	0.0 g			**Phosphorus**	175 mg

CHICKEN, ARTICHOKE, AND SPINACH SOUP

Servings: 12　　　**Serving Size:** 1 cup　　　**Prep Time:** 12 minutes　　　**Cook Time:** 45 minutes

While fresh artichokes are lovely, I really do like the frozen variety. They are so easy to toss into so many dishes. This soup is full of fiber and perfect for an autumn or winter meal.

1 tablespoon	olive oil
1 medium	onion, chopped
3	garlic cloves, minced
3/4 pound	fresh or frozen chicken breasts, thawed and patted dry, cut into 1/2-inch cubes
1 teaspoon	dried oregano
1 teaspoon	dried basil
1/4 teaspoon	crushed red pepper flakes
1/4 teaspoon	Kosher salt
1/4 teaspoon	freshly ground black pepper
5 cups	low-fat, reduced-sodium chicken broth
8 ounces	frozen yellow corn
8 ounces	frozen artichoke hearts, thawed and coarsely chopped
1 (14.5-ounce) can	no-salt-added diced tomatoes
1 (10-ounce) package	frozen chopped spinach, slightly thawed
1 tablespoon	fresh lemon juice

1. Heat the oil in a large saucepan over medium heat. Add the onion and garlic and sauté for 6–7 minutes. Add in chicken, oregano, basil, crushed red pepper, salt, and ground black pepper and sauté for about 5 minutes.

2. Add in the broth, corn, artichoke hearts, and tomatoes and bring to a boil. Lower the heat, simmer, uncovered, for 20 minutes.

3. Break up the frozen spinach into small pieces and add to the soup. Simmer 5 minutes until heated through. Add in the lemon juice and remove from the heat.

Exchanges/Choices

2 Vegetable
1 Lean Meat

Calories	90	**Cholesterol**	15 mg	**Total Carbohydrate**	9 g
Calories from Fat	20	**Sodium**	310 mg	Dietary Fiber	3 g
Total Fat	2.0 g	**Potassium**	355 mg	Sugars	3 g
Saturated Fat	0.4 g			**Protein**	9 g
Trans Fat	0.0 g			**Phosphorus**	105 mg

AROMATIC INDIAN STYLE PEA SOUP

Servings: 6	Serving Size: 1 cup	Prep Time: 8 minutes	Cook Time: 45 minutes

Minty fresh, there is nothing like pea soup enhanced with exotic spices of cumin and coriander. Frozen peas are available year round, so there's always an occasion to make this beautiful soup.

2 teaspoons	cumin seeds
1 teaspoon	coriander seeds
1 tablespoon	olive oil
1 medium	onion, diced
1 medium	leek, washed and thinly sliced (bottom white part only)
2	garlic cloves, minced
1/4 cup	fresh mint leaves
4 cups	low-fat, reduced-sodium chicken broth
1 (10-ounce) package	frozen peas, thawed
1/4 teaspoon	Kosher salt
1/4 teaspoon	freshly ground black pepper

Garnish

	fresh mint sprigs
1/2 cup	plain non-fat yogurt

1. Add the cumin and coriander seeds to a small dry skillet. Toast over medium-high heat, shaking the pan occasionally until the seeds are toasted and become aromatic, about 3–4 minutes. Remove the skillet from the heat and set aside.

2. Heat the olive oil in a large saucepan over medium-high heat. Add the onion, leek, and garlic and sauté for 6–7 minutes until tender.

3. Using a large square of cheesecloth, place the toasted cumin and coriander seeds and the mint leaves in the center of the cloth; tie the ends of the cheesecloth together to form a sachet. Add the sachet and the broth to the onion mixture and bring to a light boil. Reduce the heat; simmer on low heat for 20 minutes.

4. Remove the sachet from the soup and add the peas, salt, and pepper and simmer for 2 minutes. In batches, puree the pea soup and return to the saucepot. Garnish with a sprig of mint and a dollop of yogurt.

Exchanges/Choices

1/2 Starch	**Calories**	110	**Cholesterol**	0 mg	**Total Carbohydrate**	16 g
2 Vegetable	Calories from Fat	20	**Sodium**	475 mg	Dietary Fiber	3 g
1/2 Fat	**Total Fat**	2.5 g	**Potassium**	310 mg	Sugars	6 g
	Saturated Fat	0.4 g			**Protein**	6 g
	Trans Fat	0.0 g			**Phosphorus**	105 mg

CHAPTER 3
Treasures from the Salad Bar

I remember when my local market opened its first salad bar. It was so exciting—everyone got to construct their own salad from crisp offerings without ever having to chop, dice, or slice a thing. Back then salad bars were pretty basic: There were a few varieties of lettuce, sliced tomatoes, chopped egg, spinach, onions, croutons, and a selection of salad dressings. Today, salad bars are a bevy of goodies too delicious to pass up.

In these recipes, you'll select already cut, sliced, and diced fruits and vegetables, grains, meats, and cheeses, but if your salad bar doesn't provide a particular ingredient, you will need to get out the knife and chopping board. However, even the most basic salad bar should have most of the ingredients called for in these recipes.

Although it's just as easy to pick up canned beans from the shelf, take advantage of scooping some beans from the salad bar when you don't need a full can. I also suggest choosing Parmesan and feta cheeses if available from your salad bar. Since these can be high in fat, just taking what you need is a good lesson in portion control. I even recommend buying already cubed tofu which many salad bars display these days.

A few tips in using a salad bar for best results:

1. Always buy from a salad bar that is regularly replenished. Stand around the salad bar section and see how often they change the bins and how many people shop from the bar.

2. Make sure your salad bar has installed proper sneeze guards and that the salad bar looks clean and fresh.

3. Try to shop from the salad bar first thing in the morning when it's first filled. The vegetables will be the least exposed to light and air, which slowly destroys their nutrient content.

4. As you plan your meals, take into account how many meals will be eaten away from home. Using the salad bar is a great way to get the exact amount of vegetables you need, while avoiding the waste that often comes when we purchase whole vegetables that won't have a chance to get eaten.

5. Consider selecting vegetables from the salad bar that are a challenge to cut up whole. Vegetables such as cabbage and jicama are already cut beautifully for you and you save time and effort with less waste.

6. Don't like slicing onions? I always seek out already sliced onions on the salad bar; it saves a lot of tears!

7. Use the salad bar for the clean vegetables and fruits but avoid already prepared salad mixtures. Already prepared pasta, potato, meat, and poultry salads may look enticing, but chances are they contain a lot of fat and sodium. Use the salad bar as a tool to save preparation time only.

TOFU VEGETABLE SALAD WITH ASIAN DRESSING

Servings: 4   Serving Size: 1 cup   Prep Time: 10 minutes   Cook Time: 0

The first time I tried tofu, it was served cold. At first I wasn't sure about how uncooked tofu would taste, but when combined with bold ingredients, it shined! A nutty Asian-inspired dressing does wonders for jazzing up tofu. This pretty little salad packs up well for easy, healthy lunches.

Salad

1/2 pound	salad bar tofu cubes or extra-firm packaged tofu, cut into 1-inch cubes
1/2 cup	shredded carrots
1/2 cup	sliced red bell pepper
1/2 cup	sliced green pepper
1/2 cup	sliced red onion
1/2 cup	peas
2 tablespoons	toasted sesame seeds

Dressing

2 tablespoons	rice vinegar
1 tablespoon	fresh lime juice
1 teaspoon	honey
1/2 teaspoon	Dijon mustard
2 1/2 tablespoons	peanut oil
1/2 teaspoon	toasted sesame oil
4 cups	mixed greens

1. In a large bowl, combine the salad ingredients.

2. In a small bowl, whisk together the rice vinegar, lime juice, honey, and Dijon mustard. In a thin stream, slowly add the peanut and sesame oils and whisk until emulsified. Pour the dressing over the salad and mix gently.

3. Line a platter or shallow bowl with mixed greens. Pile the tofu salad onto the greens.

Exchanges/Choices

1/2 Starch	**Calories**	215	**Cholesterol**	0 mg	**Total Carbohydrate**	14 g	
1 Vegetable	Calories from Fat	125	**Sodium**	45 mg	Dietary Fiber	4 g	
1 Lean Meat	**Total Fat**	14.0 g	**Potassium**	295 mg	Sugars	6 g	
2 1/2 Fat	Saturated Fat	2.3 g			**Protein**	9 g	
	Trans Fat	0.0 g			**Phosphorus**	160 mg	

CHICKPEA TARTINES

Servings: 4   Serving Size: 1 tartine   Prep Time: 11 minutes

The spread for these open-faced sandwiches is similar to hummus, but lighter in taste. Piled onto dark bread with colorful carrots and tomatoes, these sandwiches are a real step up from a humdrum turkey sandwich. You can even cut these into small pieces and serve them as little appetizers.

Spread

1 cup	chickpeas
2 tablespoons	olive oil
2 tablespoons	lemon juice
2 tablespoons	chopped scallions
1	garlic clove, minced
1 tablespoon	parmesan cheese
1/4–1/2 teaspoon	hot sauce
4 slices	toasted rye or pumpernickel bread

Topping

1/2 cup	shredded carrots
4 slices	tomato

1. Combine all the ingredients for the spread in a food processor or blender and blend until smooth, but thick.

2. Divide the spread evenly over each slice of bread. Top each slice with carrots and tomatoes.

Exchanges/Choices

2 Starch	**Calories**	220	**Cholesterol**	0 mg	**Total Carbohydrate**	29 g
1 1/2 Fat	Calories from Fat	80	**Sodium**	310 mg	Dietary Fiber	5 g
	Total Fat	9.0 g	**Potassium**	270 mg	Sugars	3 g
	Saturated Fat	1.4 g			**Protein**	7 g
	Trans Fat	0.0 g			**Phosphorus**	125 mg

SIRLOIN WITH BROCCOLI AND PEPPERS

Servings: 8	Serving Size: 1 cup	Prep Time: 10 minutes	Cook Time: 10 minutes

Salad bars are a gold mine for stir-fry ingredients. This simple sirloin stir-fry gets all dressed up with red peppers, red onions, and broccoli dressing in a garlic and herb touched sauce.

1 tablespoon	vegetable oil, divided
1 pound	boneless sirloin steak, trimmed and cut into 1/2-inch strips
2	garlic cloves, minced
1 cup	sliced red onion
2 cups	sliced red bell pepper
2 cups	broccoli florets
2 tablespoons	flour
1 tablespoon	salt-free garlic and herb seasoning (such as Mrs. Dash)
2/3 cup	low-fat, reduced-sodium beef broth
1 tablespoon	tomato paste
2 teaspoons	fresh lime juice

1 Heat 1/2 tablespoon of the oil in a large wok or heavy pan. Add half the sirloin and cook for about 2–3 minutes. Remove the beef from the pan and repeat with the remaining half. Remove the beef from the pan and set aside.

2 Add the remaining oil to the pan. Add the garlic and red onion and sauté for 2 minutes. Add the red pepper and sauté for 2 minutes. Add the broccoli and sauté for 1 minute.

3 Add the flour and garlic and herb seasoning to the vegetables and cook for 1 minute.

4 Combine the broth, tomato paste, and lime juice. Add to the pan, cover, and steam for 1 minute until broccoli is bright green. Uncover and add the beef back to the pan and toss gently with vegetables and sauce.

Exchanges/Choices

1 Vegetable
2 Lean Meat

Calories	110	**Cholesterol**	20 mg	**Total Carbohydrate**	6 g
Calories from Fat	35	**Sodium**	85 mg	Dietary Fiber	1 g
Total Fat	4.0 g	**Potassium**	315 mg	Sugars	2 g
Saturated Fat	1.1 g			**Protein**	13 g
Trans Fat	0.1 g			**Phosphorus**	120 mg

VEGETABLE POLENTA

Servings: 8   Serving Size: 1 cup   Prep Time: 10 minutes   Cook Time: 36 minutes

Convenient prepared polenta marries with salad bar staples of mushrooms and peppers to create this lasagna-like dish. So comforting and homey, this is a perfect solution for a wintry night meal.

1 tablespoon	olive oil
2	garlic cloves, minced
2 tablespoons	chopped scallions
4 cups	sliced mushrooms
2 cups	sliced red bell pepper
2 teaspoon	dried oregano
1 teaspoon	dried basil
1/4 teaspoon	crushed red pepper
2 (14.5-ounce) cans	diced Italian-style tomatoes
1 tube	prepared polenta
2 tablespoons	grated fresh parmesan cheese

1. Preheat the oven to 400 degrees. Coat a 9 × 13-inch pan with cooking spray and set aside.

2. Heat the oil in a large skillet over medium heat. Add the garlic, scallions, and mushrooms and sauté for about 3 minutes. Add the red peppers and sauté for 2–3 minutes. Add in the oregano, basil, crushed red pepper, and tomatoes. Bring to a boil. Reduce the heat to low and simmer for 10 minutes.

3. Slice the polenta and place on the bottom of the prepared pan. Spread the mushroom sauce over the polenta. Cover and bake for about 15 minutes. Uncover and sprinkle with the parmesan cheese and bake for 5 minutes.

Exchanges/Choices

1/2 Starch	**Calories**	110	**Cholesterol**	0 mg	**Total Carbohydrate**	19 g
2 Vegetable	Calories from Fat	25	**Sodium**	560 mg	Dietary Fiber	2 g
1/2 Fat	**Total Fat**	3.0 g	**Potassium**	410 mg	Sugars	6 g
	Saturated Fat	0.6 g			**Protein**	4 g
	Trans Fat	0.0 g			**Phosphorus**	80 mg

CAULIFLOWER CHICKPEA CURRY

Servings: 5   **Serving Size:** 1 cup   **Prep Time:** 15 minutes   **Cook Time:** 30 minutes

Whenever I dine at Indian restaurants, I always go for something with cauliflower and chickpeas. The cuisine of India always inspires me to create assertively flavored dishes. So make use of those already cut cauliflower florets just waiting there for you to pick up at your local salad bar.

1 tablespoon	olive oil
1 cup	sliced red onion
1 cup	sliced carrots
1 1/2 cups	cauliflower florets
2	garlic cloves, minced
1 tablespoon	curry powder
1 teaspoon	brown sugar
1 teaspoon	ground ginger
1 1/4 cups	low-fat, reduced-sodium chicken broth
1 (14.5-ounce) can	diced tomatoes, drained
1 cup	canned chickpeas, drained
3/4 cup	light coconut milk

1. Heat the oil in a large wok or heavy pan over medium heat. Add the red onion and carrots and stir-fry for 3 minutes. Add in the cauliflower and garlic and stir-fry for 3 minutes. Combine the curry powder, brown sugar, and ginger and add to the vegetables, stir-fry for 1 minute.

2. Add the broth and tomatoes to the vegetables and bring to a boil. Cover, reduce the heat to low, and simmer for 15 minutes until the vegetables are tender.

3. Add in the chickpeas and coconut milk. Simmer for 1 minute.

Exchanges/Choices

1/2 Starch	**Calories**	145	**Cholesterol**	0 mg	**Total Carbohydrate**	20 g
2 Vegetable	Calories from Fat	55	**Sodium**	280 mg	Dietary Fiber	5 g
1 Fat	**Total Fat**	6.0 g	**Potassium**	520 mg	Sugars	7 g
	Saturated Fat	2.4 g			**Protein**	6 g
	Trans Fat	0.0 g			**Phosphorus**	135 mg

SALAD BAR SALSA WITH GRILLED FLANK STEAK

Servings: 4   **Serving Size:** 3 ounces, 1/3 cup salsa   **Prep Time:** 15 minutes   **Cook Time:** 8 minutes

Salsa isn't just tomatoes. Scour the salad bar and you'll find a bevy of ingredients to make homemade salsa special. Paired with a juicy, but lean grilled steak, it's a perfect summer meal.

Salsa

1 cup	yellow corn
1 cup	quartered cherry tomatoes
1/4 cup	diced red onion
2 tablespoons	minced scallions
3 tablespoons	fresh lime juice
1/2 tablespoon	olive oil
1/4 teaspoon	cayenne pepper
1/4 teaspoon	sugar

Steak

1 pound	flank steak
2 teaspoons	paprika
1 teaspoon	chili powder
1/2 teaspoon	Kosher salt
1/4 teaspoon	freshly ground black pepper
1 tablespoon	olive oil

1. In a medium bowl, combine all the ingredients for the salsa. Set aside.

2. Trim any excess fat from the flank steak. Using a sharp knife, make 3 diagonal slashes across the top surface of the steak, cutting about 1/3 of the way through the steak. This will prevent it from curling up on the grill.

3. Preheat the grill to medium-high heat. Coat the grill rack with cooking spray or prepare an oven broiler. Cover a broiler pan with foil. Coat the foil with cooking spray. Combine the paprika, chili powder, salt, and pepper. Brush both sides of the steak with the olive oil. Sprinkle both sides with the spice mixture. Grill the steak, about 4–6 inches from the heat source, for about 5 minutes per side or until desired doneness.

4. Remove the steak from the oven onto a carving board. Let the steak stand for 5 minutes before slicing. Cut the steak diagonally across the grain into thin slices. Serve with the salsa.

Exchanges/Choices

1/2 Starch	**Calories**	245	**Cholesterol**	40 mg	**Total Carbohydrate**	12 g
1 Vegetable	Calories from Fat	110	**Sodium**	180 mg	Dietary Fiber	2 g
3 Lean Meat	**Total Fat**	12.0 g	**Potassium**	530 mg	Sugars	3 g
1 Fat	Saturated Fat	3.3 g			**Protein**	24 g
	Trans Fat	0.0 g			**Phosphorus**	220 mg

SALAD BAR OMELETTE

Serving: 1   Serving Size: 1 omelette   Prep Time: 15 minutes   Cook Time: 10 minutes

Omelets are great anytime. And with a quick stop at the salad bar, you can load your omelet up with great veggies, such as mushrooms, spinach, and cherry tomatoes. Forget about gobs of cheese in this omelet; all it needs is a very light touch of feta.

	cooking spray
2 teaspoons	non-hydrogenated spread, such as Smart Balance
1/2 cup	sliced mushrooms
1 cup	baby spinach leaves
1/4 cup	halved cherry tomatoes
1/2 cup	egg substitute
1 tablespoon	fat-free milk
	dash hot sauce
	dash Kosher salt
1/8 teaspoon	freshly ground black pepper
1 teaspoon	crumbled feta cheese

1 Coat a nonstick skillet with cooking spray. Add the spread to the skillet and turn the heat to medium high. Add in the mushrooms and sauté for about 5 minutes until golden. Add in the spinach and cherry tomatoes and sauté just until the spinach wilts and before it releases too much liquid. Remove the vegetable mixture from the pan.

2 Wipe the skillet clean and coat with cooking spray. Mix together the egg substitute, milk, and hot sauce. Add the egg mixture to the skillet and cook over medium heat undisturbed for 30 seconds. Using a thin bladed spatula, push the edges of the eggs toward the center. Cook until the eggs are moist but no longer runny.

3 Add the vegetable mixture across one side of the omelet and using a large spatula, fold the omelet in half. Let the omelet cook 1 minute. Slip the omelet out of the pan onto a plate and sprinkle with feta cheese.

Exchanges/Choices

1 Vegetable	**Calories**	155	**Cholesterol**	5 mg	**Total Carbohydrate**	8 g
2 Lean Meat	Calories from Fat	65	**Sodium**	495 mg	Dietary Fiber	2 g
1/2 Fat	**Total Fat**	7.0 g	**Potassium**	740 mg	Sugars	4 g
	Saturated Fat	2.2 g			**Protein**	16 g
	Trans Fat	0.0 g			**Phosphorus**	110 mg

VIETNAMESE CABBAGE AND PORK SALAD

Servings: 8   **Serving Size:** 1 cup   **Prep Time:** 20 minutes   **Cook Time:** 25 minutes

I love that salad bars are now adding fresh sliced cabbage to the bins. It's so much easier to have pre-sliced cabbage on hand to create this refreshing summer salad. Use this dressing also as a marinade for other foods such as chicken or beef.

1 pound	pork tenderloin
1 teaspoon	olive oil
1/4 teaspoon	Kosher salt
1/4 teaspoon	freshly ground black pepper

Salad

2 cups	sliced green cabbage
1/2 cup	thinly sliced red onion
1/2 cup	sliced cucumber

Dressing

3 tablespoons	fresh lime juice
1 tablespoons	fish sauce
1 tablespoon	lite soy sauce
1 teaspoon	sesame oil
1/2 teaspoon	sugar
1/8 teaspoon	cayenne pepper

4 cups	torn romaine lettuce leaves

1. Preheat the oven to 400 degrees. Cover a broiler rack with foil. Coat the foil with cooking spray. Rub the pork with the oil, salt, and pepper. Roast the pork for about 20 minutes. Turn the oven to broil and broil the pork for about 5 minutes, turning once until a meat thermometer registers 145 degrees when inserted into the thickest part of the pork. Remove the pork from the oven to a carving board and let rest.

2. In a large bowl, combine the cabbage, red onion, and cucumber. Whisk together the lime juice, fish sauce, soy sauce, sesame oil, sugar, and cayenne pepper. Add to the cabbage mixture and toss well. Cut the pork into thin slices and add to the salad and toss again.

3. Line a platter with romaine lettuce. Pile the pork salad on top of the lettuce.

Exchanges/Choices

1 Vegetable	**Calories**	85	**Cholesterol**	30 mg	**Total Carbohydrate**	4 g
1 Lean Meat	Calories from Fat	20	**Sodium**	325 mg	Dietary Fiber	1 g
1/2 Fat	**Total Fat**	2.5 g	**Potassium**	305 mg	Sugars	2 g
	Saturated Fat	0.7 g			**Protein**	12 g
	Trans Fat	0.0 g			**Phosphorus**	120 mg

SALAD BAR PIZZA

Servings: 8   **Serving Size:** 1 slice   **Prep Time:** 5 minutes   **Cook Time:** 45 minutes

Make your own pizza at home. It's easy to load up on a bevy of vegetable toppings when you utilize the salad bar! With readymade dough, you can have a healthy veggie-filled pizza in less time than delivery.

2 tablespoons plus 1 teaspoon	olive oil, divided
3 cups	sliced mushrooms
2 cups	sliced red pepper
1 cup	sliced red onion
3	garlic cloves, thinly sliced
1 teaspoon	dried oregano
1/2 teaspoon	dried basil
1/4 teaspoon	crushed red pepper flakes
1 pound	fresh pizza dough, preferably whole-wheat
1 tablespoon	cornmeal
2 ounces	shredded part-skim mozzarella cheese
1/4 cup	fresh grated parmesan cheese
1 cup	cherry tomatoes, halved

1. Preheat the oven to 450 degrees. Heat 1 tablespoon of the oil in a large skillet. Add the mushrooms and cook undisturbed for 2 minutes. Stir the mushrooms and cook for about 4 minutes until golden brown. Remove from the skillet and add to a bowl.

2. Add another tablespoon of oil to the pan. Add the red peppers and red onion and sauté for 5 minutes. Add in the garlic, oregano, basil, and crushed red pepper flakes and sauté for 1 minute. Add to the mushrooms.

3. Roll the dough into a large circle on a lightly floured surface. Sprinkle a large pizza pan with cornmeal. Place the dough on the pan. Brush the surface of the dough with the 1 teaspoon olive oil. Sprinkle the dough with the mozzarella cheese. Top with the vegetable mixture. Sprinkle with the Parmesan cheese.

4. Bake the pizza for about 20 minutes or until golden brown. Add the cherry tomatoes to the pizza and bake another 5 minutes. Remove from the oven, let rest for a few minutes, and cut into slices.

Exchanges/Choices

1 1/2 Starch	**Calories**	210	**Cholesterol**	5 mg	
1 Vegetable	Calories from Fat	70	**Sodium**	320 mg	
1 1/2 Fat	**Total Fat**	8.0 g	**Potassium**	325 mg	
	Saturated Fat	1.9 g			
	Trans Fat	0.0 g			

Total Carbohydrate	30 g
Dietary Fiber	3 g
Sugars	3 g
Protein	8 g
Phosphorus	190 mg

ROASTED SHRIMP WITH CABBAGE SLAW

Servings: 6   Serving Size: 1 cup   Prep Time: 15 minutes   Cook Time: 7–9 minutes

We often sauté shrimp, but how about roasting them. The dry heat roasts these shrimp to perfection; they are perfectly juicy and flavorful. With ready-made veggies from the salad bar, a cool vegetable slaw accompanies these nicely spiced shrimp.

1 pound	peeled and deveined large shrimp
2 teaspoons	salt-free Caribbean-style seasoning (such as Mrs. Dash)
2 cups	sliced green cabbage
1 cup	sliced red cabbage
1/2 cup	sliced or shredded carrots
1/2 cup	sliced red onion
2 tablespoons	sliced scallions
2 tablespoons	lime juice
1 teaspoon	Dijon mustard
1/2 teaspoon	sugar
	dash hot sauce
1/4 cup	canola oil
1/4 teaspoon	Kosher salt
1/4 teaspoon	freshly ground black pepper

1 Preheat the oven to 400 degrees. Add the shrimp to a bowl. Add in the seasoning and toss to coat well. Line a broiler pan with foil. Coat the foil with cooking spray. Roast the shrimp for about 7–9 minutes until cooked through. Remove from the oven and keep warm.

2 In a medium bowl, combine the cabbages, carrot, red onion, and scallions. In a small bowl, whisk together the lime juice, mustard, sugar, and hot sauce. Slowly in a thin stream, add the oil until the dressing is emulsified. Season with salt and pepper. Pour the dressing on the cabbage salad and toss to coat. Serve the roasted shrimp with the cabbage slaw.

Exchanges/Choices

1 Vegetable	**Calories**	185	**Cholesterol**	120 mg	**Total Carbohydrate**	6 g
2 Lean Meat	Calories from Fat	90	**Sodium**	310 mg	Dietary Fiber	2 g
1 1/2 Fat	**Total Fat**	10.0 g	**Potassium**	305 mg	Sugars	3 g
	Saturated Fat	0.9 g			**Protein**	17 g
	Trans Fat	0.0 g			**Phosphorus**	185 mg

CHICKEN PENNE TARRAGON SALAD

Servings: 4   **Serving Size:** 1 cup

I make this salad every summer for our outdoor concert series. Loaded with fresh vegetables and precooked chicken, everyone around the picnic table enjoys this so much. I can't ever make anything else for my crowd!

4 ounces	whole-wheat spirals
1 cup	broccoli florets, cut into bite-sized pieces
1/2 cup	sliced red pepper
1/2 cup	sliced carrots
1 1/2 cups	cooked shredded or diced skinless white meat rotisserie chicken
1/2 cup	diced red onion
2 tablespoons	finely chopped fresh tarragon

Dressing

2 tablespoons	lemon juice or red wine vinegar
2 teaspoons	Dijon mustard
1	garlic clove, finely minced
1/2 teaspoon	sugar
3 tablespoons	olive oil
1/4 teaspoon	Kosher salt
1/4 teaspoon	freshly ground black pepper

Garnish

1 1/2 tablespoons	crumbled blue cheese

1. Cook the pasta according to package directions. Add in the broccoli, red pepper, and carrots during the last 2 minutes of cooking. Drain and rinse lightly with cold water. Drain again.

2. Add the pasta and vegetables to a bowl. Add in the chicken, red onion, and tarragon and toss.

3. In a small bowl, whisk together the lemon juice, mustard, garlic, and sugar. Slowly, in a thin stream, whisk in the olive oil until emulsified. Season with salt and pepper. Add the dressing to the salad. Add in the blue cheese and mix.

Exchanges/Choices

1 1/2 Starch
1 Vegetable
2 Lean Meat
2 Fat

Calories	315	**Cholesterol**	50 mg	**Total Carbohydrate**	28 g
Calories from Fat	125	**Sodium**	425 mg	Dietary Fiber	5 g
Total Fat	14.0 g	**Potassium**	385 mg	Sugars	4 g
Saturated Fat	2.5 g			**Protein**	22 g
Trans Fat	0.1 g			**Phosphorus**	240 mg

GRILLED VEGETABLE SANDWICH

Change up from the usual meat-based sandwiches to something truly more healthful. With salad bar veggies just begging to be grilled, this sandwich is so good you might just dump the typical turkey sandwich in favor of this creation.

1 cup	zucchini slices
1 cup	yellow squash slices
1 cup	red pepper slices
3 tablespoons	reduced-fat balsamic vinaigrette
1	garlic clove, minced
	cooking spray
2 tablespoons	prepared pesto
4 slices	whole-grain bread
4 tablespoons	freshly shredded reduced-fat cheddar cheese

1. Add the zucchini, yellow squash, and red pepper slices to a large bowl. Add in the balsamic dressing and garlic and toss well.

2. Coat a grill pan with cooking spray. Add the vegetables and grill for about 4–5 minutes on each side until tender.

3. Set an oven broiler to high. Set the rack about 4–6 inches from the heat source. Line a baking sheet with foil. Spread each slice of bread with pesto. Evenly distribute the grilled vegetables among the bread slices. Top with 1 tablespoon of cheese. Add the bread slices to the prepared baking sheet. Broil the sandwiches just until the cheese melts, about 2–3 minutes.

Exchanges/Choices

1 Starch	**Calories**	135	**Cholesterol**	5 mg	**Total Carbohydrate**	17 g
1 Fat	Calories from Fat	55	**Sodium**	365 mg	Dietary Fiber	3 g
	Total Fat	6.0 g	**Potassium**	285 mg	Sugars	3 g
	Saturated Fat	1.5 g			**Protein**	6 g
	Trans Fat	0.0 g			**Phosphorus**	140 mg

BLACK BEAN TACOS

Servings: 4   Serving Size: 1 taco   Prep Time: 5 minutes   Cook Time: 18 minutes

One of my testers said her family ate these with such gusto, she couldn't keep up with the demand for more! With red onion slices and a scoop of black beans from the salad bar, these fresh tacos might have your family begging for more!

1 tablespoon	olive oil
1 cup	red onion slices
1 teaspoon	cumin
1/2 teaspoon	chili powder
1/4 teaspoon	dried oregano
1/4 teaspoon	Kosher salt
1/4 teaspoon	freshly ground black pepper
1 cup	black beans (from the salad bar or canned, drained and rinsed)
1/2 cup	hot or mild salsa
1/2 cup	chopped tomato
4 (6-inch)	corn tortillas

Garnish

1/2 cup	plain, non-fat yogurt or non-fat sour cream
	fresh lime wedges

1. Heat the oil in a large skillet over medium-high heat. Add the red onions, lower the heat to medium, and sauté for about 5–6 minutes. Lower the heat to medium low, add the cumin, chili powder, oregano, salt, and pepper and sauté for 3–4 minutes. Set aside.

2. In a medium bowl, mix together the black beans and salsa. Set aside.

3. Heat a large skillet over medium-high heat. Add tortillas, one at a time, and cook on each side for about 1–2 minutes until soft and warmed.

4. Divide the bean salsa mixture among the tortillas. Top with the sautéed onions and chopped tomato.

5. Garnish with yogurt or sour cream. Squeeze lime on top.

Exchanges/Choices

1 1/2 Starch
1 Vegetable
1 Fat

Calories	180	**Cholesterol**	0 mg	**Total Carbohydrate**	30 g
Calories from Fat	40	**Sodium**	390 mg	Dietary Fiber	6 g
Total Fat	4.5 g	**Potassium**	465 mg	Sugars	6 g
Saturated Fat	0.7 g			**Protein**	8 g
Trans Fat	0.0 g			**Phosphorus**	210 mg

ITALIAN SHRIMP, BEAN, AND VEGETABLE SALAD

Servings: 4 Serving Size: 1 cup Prep Time: 15 minutes Cook Time: 0

They say we eat with our eyes and nothing could be truer when you gaze upon this colorful healthy main dish salad. Select pretty hues from the salad bar, toss in some shrimp, and whip up a basil-touched dressing and you've got a fantastic light meal.

10 ounces	fresh cooked shrimp, cut into bite-sized pieces
1 cup	halved cherry tomatoes
1 cup	chickpeas (from salad bar or canned, drained and rinsed)
1/2 cup	sliced carrots
1/2 cup	sliced red onion
2 tablespoons	sliced scallions

Dressing

2 tablespoons	fresh lemon juice
1 teaspoon	Dijon mustard
1/2 teaspoon	dried oregano
1/2 teaspoon	dried basil
1/2 teaspoon	sugar
1	garlic clove, finely minced
3 tablespoons	olive oil
1/4 teaspoon	Kosher salt
1/4 teaspoon	freshly ground black pepper
4 cups	baby spinach leaves

Garnish

2 tablespoons	chopped pitted black olives

1 In a large bowl, combine the shrimp, cherry tomatoes, chickpeas, carrots, red onion, and scallions.

2 In a small bowl, whisk together the lemon juice, mustard, oregano, basil, sugar, and garlic. Slowly, in a thin stream, whisk in the olive oil until emulsified. Season with salt and pepper. Pour over the shrimp and vegetables. Serve over spinach leaves and garnish with olives.

Exchanges/Choices

1/2 Starch	**Calories**	285	**Cholesterol**	150 mg	**Total Carbohydrate**	21 g
2 Vegetable	Calories from Fat	115	**Sodium**	510 mg	Dietary Fiber	6 g
3 Lean Meat	**Total Fat**	13.0 g	**Potassium**	755 mg	Sugars	6 g
1 1/2 Fat	Saturated Fat	2.0 g			**Protein**	22 g
	Trans Fat	0.0 g			**Phosphorus**	335 mg

SEARED CHERRY TOMATO, PEA, AND RED PEPPER PASTA

Servings: 8   Serving Size: 1 cup   Prep Time: 20 minutes   Cook Time: 17 minutes

Cherry tomatoes taste so rich when lightly seared in a pan. Fortunately, the salad bar is always stocked with fresh ones, so this colorful main dish can be a dinner mainstay. Toss in salad bar red peppers and some green peas and you have a hearty, healthy, fiber-filled meal.

8 ounces	thin spaghetti (preferably whole-wheat)
2 tablespoons	olive oil
1/2 cup	sliced red bell pepper
2 cups	halved cherry tomatoes
2 tablespoons	dried breadcrumbs
3	garlic cloves, thinly sliced
1/2 cup	green peas
1/2 teaspoon	salt-free dried Italian seasoning
	pinch crushed red pepper flakes
2 tablespoons	fresh grated Parmesan cheese

1. Cook the spaghetti according to package directions.

2. Meanwhile, heat 1 tablespoon of the oil in a large skillet. Add the red pepper and sauté for 2 minutes. Add the cherry tomatoes and sauté until seared, about 2 minutes. Sprinkle with breadcrumbs and toss to coat. Remove the pepper-cherry mixture from the skillet and set aside.

3. Add the remaining oil to the pan and cook the garlic for 30 seconds. Add the peas, Italian seasoning, and red pepper flakes and cook for 1 minute.

4. Drain the pasta, reserving 1/2 cup of the cooking water. Add the pasta and reserved water to the garlic-pea mixture. Add the cherry tomato mixture to the pasta and mix well. Toss with Parmesan cheese and serve.

Exchanges/Choices

1 1/2 Starch
1 Fat

Calories	165	**Cholesterol**	0 mg	**Total Carbohydrate**	25 g
Calories from Fat	40	Sodium	40 mg	Dietary Fiber	4 g
Total Fat	4.5 g	Potassium	165 mg	Sugars	2 g
Saturated Fat	0.8 g			**Protein**	6 g
Trans Fat	0.0 g			**Phosphorus**	85 mg

SALAD BAR GAZPACHO SALAD

Servings: 5   Serving Size: 1 cup   Prep Time: 10 minutes

One of my favorite soups of all time is cool gazpacho. I just love the fresh flavors and thought, "Why not reach beyond gazpacho as a soup and turn it into a salad!" With all ready-cut veggies from the salad bar, all the labor is done!

2 cups	chickpeas, red kidney beans, or black beans (from salad bar or canned, drained and rinsed)
1 1/2 cups	diced tomatoes
2/3 cup	corn
2/3 cup	diced cucumber
3 tablespoons	diced red onion
2 tablespoons	minced cilantro
1/4 cup	low-sodium tomato juice
2 tablespoons	fresh lime juice
1 tablespoon	olive oil
1/2 teaspoon	mild or hot chili powder
1/4 teaspoon	salt
1/4 teaspoon	freshly ground black pepper
5 cups	mixed greens

1. Combine the beans, tomato, corn, cucumber, red onion, and cilantro.

2. In a small bowl, whisk together the tomato juice, lime juice, olive oil, chili powder, salt, and pepper. Pour over the salad and mix gently. Serve over mixed greens.

Exchanges/Choices

1 Starch	**Calories**	160	**Cholesterol**	0 mg	**Total Carbohydrate**	25 g
1 Vegetable	Calories from Fat	40	**Sodium**	230 mg	Dietary Fiber	6 g
1 Fat	**Total Fat**	4.5 g	**Potassium**	420 mg	Sugars	6 g
	Saturated Fat	0.6 g			**Protein**	7 g
	Trans Fat	0.0 g			**Phosphorus**	140 mg

BEANS AND GREENS WITH WHOLE-WHEAT SHELLS

Servings: 8   Serving Size: 1 cup   Prep Time: 10 minutes   Cook Time: 7–8 minutes

Probably the fastest recipe in the book, hot pasta "cooks" salad bar spinach ever so lightly to preserve texture and nutrition. Toss in some salad bar chickpeas and you have a speedy dinner perfect for rushed nights.

8 ounces	whole-wheat shells
8 cups	salad bar spinach leaves, stems removed
2 cups	chickpeas (from salad bar or canned, rinsed and drained)
1/4 cup	grated Pecorino Romano cheese
2 tablespoons	olive oil
1/2 teaspoon	salt-free garlic and herb seasoning (such as Mrs. Dash)
1/4 teaspoon	freshly ground black pepper

1. Prepare the whole-wheat shells according to package directions.

2. Add the spinach, chickpeas, cheese, olive oil, garlic seasoning, and black pepper to a large bowl. Drain the pasta but do not rinse. Immediately add the hot pasta to the spinach mixture and mix well until the spinach wilts slightly.

Exchanges/Choices

2 Starch	**Calories**	205	**Cholesterol**	5 mg	**Total Carbohydrate**	33 g
1 Lean Meat	Calories from Fat	55	**Sodium**	125 mg	Dietary Fiber	6 g
	Total Fat	6.0 g	**Potassium**	320 mg	Sugars	3 g
	Saturated Fat	1.1 g			**Protein**	9 g
	Trans Fat	0.0 g			**Phosphorus**	170 mg

SALAD BAR ROASTED VEGETABLE SALAD

Salad bar offerings go from cold to bold! Why not take the usual salad bar ingredients and cook them up in this lovely vegetarian main dish salad. There is a world beyond just using the salad bar for "salad" and this recipe shows how to bring out the fabulous flavors in your salad bar favorites.

2 cups	sliced mushrooms
2 cups	sliced carrots
2 cups	chopped yellow peppers
2 cups	halved cherry tomatoes
1/2 cup	coarsely chopped onion
1 1/2 tablespoons	olive oil
1 tablespoon	balsamic vinegar
1/2 teaspoon	dried oregano
1/2 teaspoon	Kosher salt
1/4 teaspoon	freshly ground black pepper
1/4 cup	chopped pitted Kalamata olives
2 cups	chickpeas
6 cups	spinach leaves

1. Preheat the oven to 400 degrees. Line 2 baking sheets with nonstick foil or parchment paper.

2. In a large bowl, combine all ingredients except the olives, chickpeas and spinach. Divide the mixture between the two baking sheets in a single layer.

3. Roast the vegetables for about 20 minutes, stirring once until vegetables are soft and golden brown.

4. Add the roasted vegetables to a bowl. Mix in the chickpeas, and olives. Serve the salad warm over fresh spinach leaves.

Exchanges/Choices

1 Starch	**Calories**	190	**Cholesterol**	0 mg	**Total Carbohydrate**	26 g	
2 Vegetable	Calories from Fat	65	**Sodium**	375 mg	Dietary Fiber	7 g	
1 1/2 Fat	**Total Fat**	7.0 g	**Potassium**	625 mg	Sugars	9 g	
	Saturated Fat	0.9 g			**Protein**	7 g	
	Trans Fat	0.0 g			**Phosphorus**	150 mg	

Roast Beef Rollups, page 65

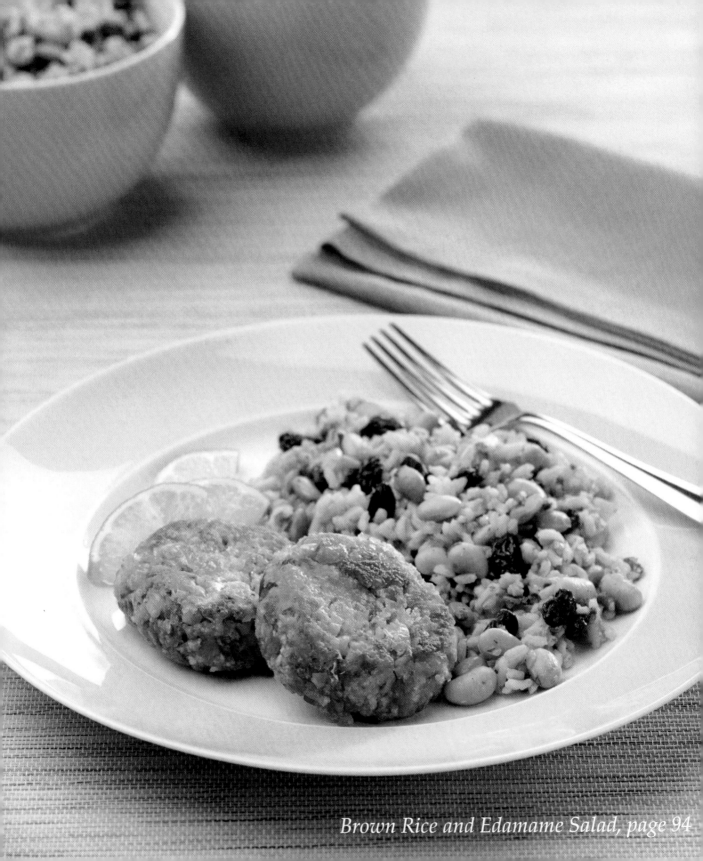

Brown Rice and Edamame Salad, page 94

Rigatoni with Sun-Dried Tomatoes, Pesto, and Olives, page 117

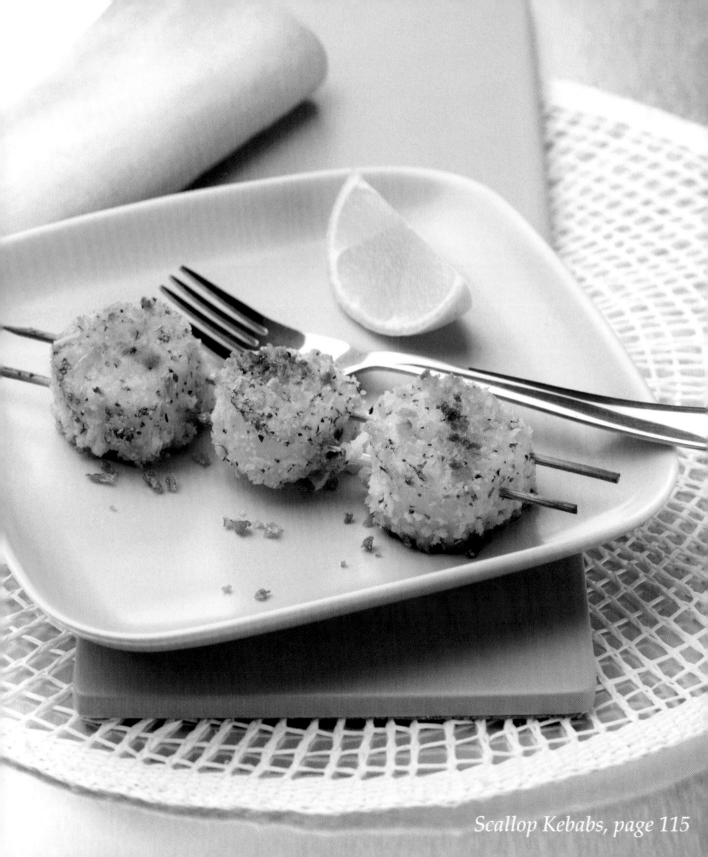

Scallop Kebabs, page 115

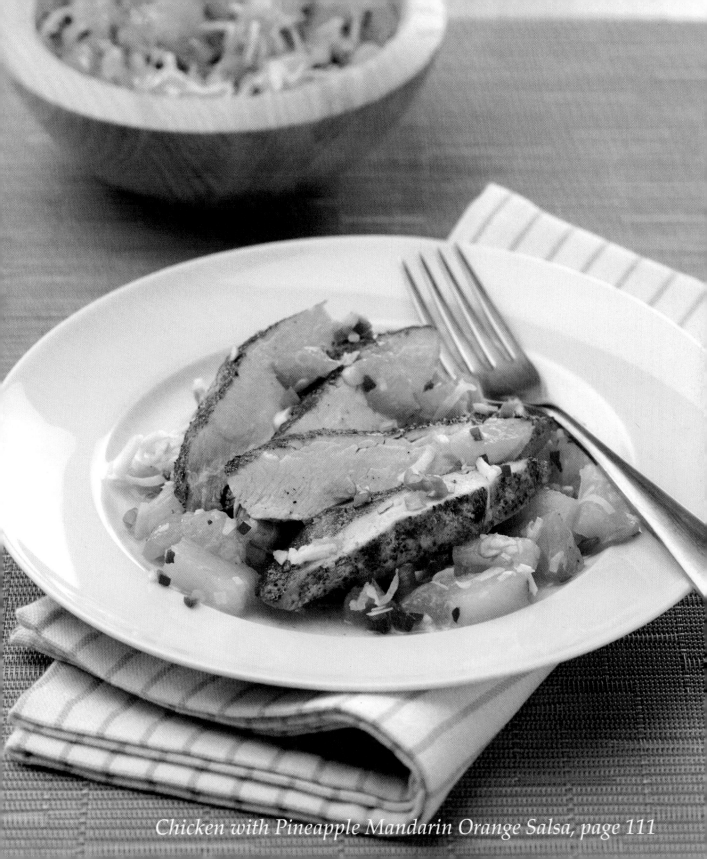

Chicken with Pineapple Mandarin Orange Salsa, page 111

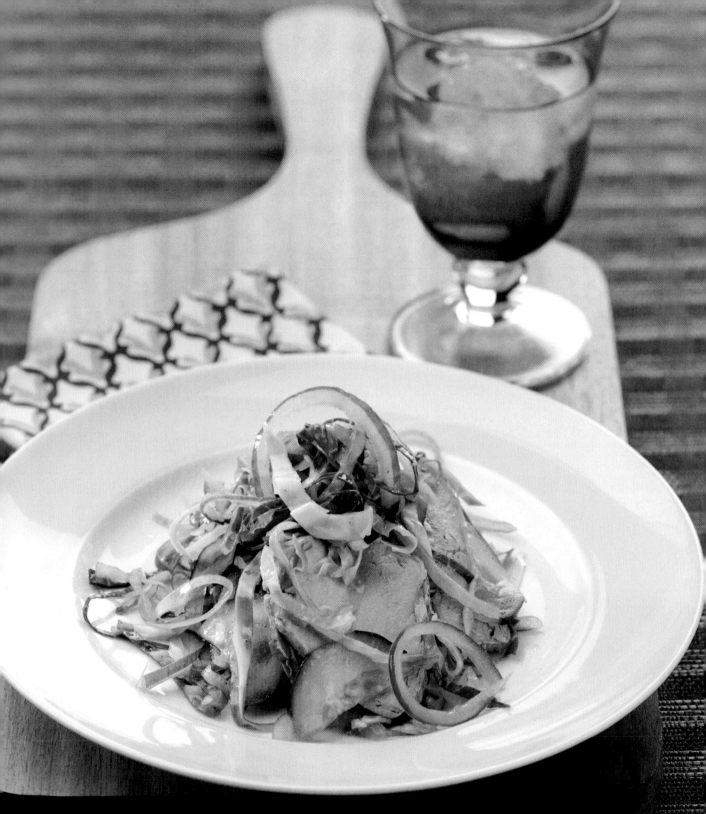

Vietnamese Cabbage and Pork Salad, page 42

Ginger Honeydew Soup, page 28

Shrimp and Bell Pepper Tacos, page 82; Melon Coolers, page 147

ISRAELI COUSCOUS WITH DOUBLE PEAS

Servings: 4   **Serving Size:** 1 cup   **Prep Time:** 25 minutes   **Cook Time:** 10 minutes

Salad bar chickpeas, cucumbers, green peas, red pepper, and scallions get tossed with fabulous easy-to-cook Israeli couscous. This super healthy main dish benefits from both fiber-rich green peas and chickpeas. Their soft textures blend beautifully with the crunchy vegetables. A light citrus dressing infused with aromatic cinnamon and cardamom completes this dish.

1 teaspoon	olive oil
1/4 cup	chopped onion
1 cup	Israeli couscous
1 1/2 cups	water
1 cup	chickpeas (from salad bar or canned, drained and rinsed)
1/2 cup	diced cucumber
1/2 cup	green peas (fresh or frozen, thawed)
1/2 cup	diced red pepper
1/4 cup	chopped parsley
2 tablespoons	chopped scallions

Dressing

3 tablespoons	orange juice
1 tablespoon	lemon juice
1/2 teaspoon	honey
1/2 teaspoon	Kosher salt
1/4 teaspoon	freshly ground black pepper

1/8 teaspoon	ground cinnamon
1/8 teaspoon	ground cardamom
2 tablespoons	olive oil

1. Heat the 1 teaspoon oil in a large skillet over medium heat. Add the onion and sauté for 3 minutes. Add the couscous and sauté for 2 minutes. Add the water and bring to a boil. Lower the heat, cover, and simmer on low heat for about 10–12 minutes or until all the water is absorbed. Add the cooked couscous to a salad bowl and let cool.

2. When the couscous has cooled to room temperature, add the chickpeas, cucumber, green peas, red pepper, parsley, and scallions, and mix well.

3. In a small bowl, whisk together the orange juice, lemon juice, honey, salt, pepper, cinnamon, and cardamom. Slowly in a thin stream, whisk in the olive oil until emulsified. Pour the dressing over the couscous and serve.

Exchanges/Choices

3 Starch	**Calories**	315	**Cholesterol**	0 mg	**Total Carbohydrate**	48 g
1 1/2 Fat	Calories from Fat	80	**Sodium**	315 mg	Dietary Fiber	6 g
	Total Fat	9.0 g	**Potassium**	375 mg	Sugars	7 g
	Saturated Fat	1.3 g			**Protein**	10 g
	Trans Fat	0.0 g			**Phosphorus**	135 mg

SALAD BAR SUMMER PICNIC SALAD

Servings: 4   **Serving Size:** 1 cup   **Prep Time:** 10 minutes   **Cook Time:** 15 minutes

On your way to a picnic in a few hours? Stop by the salad bar and pick up practically everything you need for this light as a feather salad. To lighten up the dressing, I use non-fat yogurt and a nice spritz of lemon to make this salad cool and tangy.

4 ounces	whole-wheat elbow macaroni
1 cup	halved cherry tomatoes
2/3 cup	corn kernels
1/2 cup	green peas
1/2 cup	shredded carrots
1/4 cup	sliced scallions

Dressing

1/4 cup	low-fat mayonnaise
1/4 cup	plain non-fat yogurt
1 tablespoon	fresh lemon juice or red wine vinegar
1 tablespoon	olive oil
1/2 teaspoon	Kosher salt
1/4 teaspoon	freshly ground black pepper

1. Cook the elbow macaroni according to package directions. Drain and rinse with cool water.

2. Mix the macaroni with the cherry tomatoes, corn, peas, carrots, and scallions.

3. In a small bowl, whisk together the mayonnaise, yogurt, lemon juice, olive oil, salt, and pepper. Pour over the salad and mix well.

Exchanges/Choices

2 Starch	**Calories**	200	**Cholesterol**	0 mg	**Total Carbohydrate**	35 g
1 Vegetable	Calories from Fat	45	**Sodium**	395 mg	Dietary Fiber	5 g
1/2 Fat	**Total Fat**	5.0 g	**Potassium**	345 mg	Sugars	6 g
	Saturated Fat	0.8 g			**Protein**	7 g
	Trans Fat	0.0 g			**Phosphorus**	155 mg

SALAD BAR PUTTANESCA

Servings: 4   Serving Size: 1 cup   Prep Time: 15 minutes   Cook Time: 21 minutes

Traditional puttanesca recipes can take hours to prepare. With salad bar sliced zucchini and yellow squash and a good-quality prepared marinara sauce, the workload is relieved! Use this puttanesca sauce over grilled chicken and fish as well.

1 tablespoon	olive oil
1/2 cup	diced onion
1 cup	sliced zucchini
1 cup	sliced yellow squash
1 teaspoon	dried oregano
1 teaspoon	dried basil
1 cup	commercially prepared low-sodium marinara sauce (such as Amy's or Walnut Acres)
1 1/2 teaspoons	anchovy paste
1/4 cup	pitted oil-cured black olives
2 teaspoons	capers
4 cups	cooked whole-wheat penne noodles

1. Heat the oil in a large skillet over medium-high heat. Add the onion and sauté for 3–4 minutes. Add the zucchini and yellow squash and sauté for 5 minutes. Add in the oregano and basil.

2. Add in marinara sauce, lower the heat, and simmer for 10 minutes. Add in the anchovy paste, olives, and capers and simmer for 3 minutes. Serve over hot cooked penne noodles.

Exchanges/Choices

2 1/2 Starch	**Calories**	300	**Cholesterol**	0 mg	**Total Carbohydrate**	45 g
1 Vegetable	Calories from Fat	90	**Sodium**	595 mg	Dietary Fiber	7 g
1 1/2 Fat	**Total Fat**	10.0 g	**Potassium**	425 mg	Sugars	6 g
	Saturated Fat	1.2 g			**Protein**	8 g
	Trans Fat	0.0 g			**Phosphorus**	135 mg

SALAD BAR CHERRY TOMATO SALSA WITH SEARED CHICKEN

Servings: 4   **Serving Size:** 3 oz chicken, 1/2 cup salsa   **Prep Time:** 15 minutes   **Cook Time:** 12 minutes

Although bottled salsa is readily available, why not make a quick, fresh salsa utilizing your salad bar offerings? Scoop up some cherry tomatoes, red onions, red peppers, and toss in some fresh lime juice and hot peppers and you have a quick topper for succulent seared chicken. Use this salsa for pairing with low-fat tortilla chips too!

Salsa

16	cherry tomatoes, quartered
1/2 cup	chopped red onion
1/2 cup	diced red bell pepper
2 tablespoons	minced cilantro
2	garlic cloves, minced
1 small	jalapeño pepper, seeded and diced
1/4 cup	lime juice
1/4 teaspoon	sea salt
1/4 teaspoon	freshly ground black pepper

Chicken

1 tablespoon	garlic-flavored olive oil
4 (4-ounce)	boneless skinless chicken cutlets
1/4 teaspoon	Kosher salt
1/4 teaspoon	freshly ground black pepper

1 Combine all the ingredients for the salsa in a medium bowl, cover, and set aside.

2 Meanwhile, heat the oil in a large skillet over medium-high heat. Sprinkle the chicken with salt and pepper and sear the chicken on both sides for about 5–6 minutes per side or until the chicken is cooked through. Serve a cutlet with a serving of salsa on top.

Exchanges/Choices

2 Vegetable	**Calories**	190	**Cholesterol**	65 mg	**Total Carbohydrate**	8 g
3 Lean Meat	Calories from Fat	55	**Sodium**	330 mg	Dietary Fiber	2 g
	Total Fat	6.0 g	**Potassium**	455 mg	Sugars	4 g
	Saturated Fat	1.3 g			**Protein**	25 g
	Trans Fat	0.0 g			**Phosphorus**	210 mg

SALAD BAR EGG WHITE FRITTATA

Servings: 4   Serving Size: 1/4 of frittata   Prep Time: 15 minutes   Cook Time: 20 minutes

Frittatas make any brunch table special. This one-skillet method makes it a breeze to prepare and serve. With a few offerings from the salad bar and healthy egg whites, this frittata is an inexpensive way to delight your morning guests.

1 tablespoon	olive oil
1/2 cup	chopped red onion
1/2 cup	diced red bell pepper
1/2 cup	broccoli florets
1/2 cup	diced or sliced zucchini
1 teaspoon	dried salt-free Italian seasoning
8	egg whites, beaten
1 tablespoon	fat-free milk
1/2 teaspoon	hot sauce
1/4 cup	grated Parmesan cheese

1. Heat the oil in a large ovenproof skillet over medium heat. Add the onion and sauté for 3 minutes. Add the red pepper, broccoli, and zucchini and sauté for 3–4 minutes until soft. Add in the Italian seasoning and sauté for 2 minutes.

2. Combine the egg whites, milk, and hot sauce in a bowl and whisk well. Pour the egg white mixture over the vegetables and let cook over medium heat for about 7–8 minutes or until the egg whites look almost set on the bottom. The top should be just a bit runny.

3. Set the oven to broil. Sprinkle the frittata with the cheese. Broil the frittata about 6 inches from the heat source until the eggs are set and the top is lightly browned, watching carefully so the frittata does not burn. Cut into wedges to serve.

Exchanges/Choices

1 Vegetable	**Calories**	95	**Cholesterol**	0 mg	**Total Carbohydrate**	5 g	
1 Lean Meat	Calories from Fat	40	**Sodium**	160 mg	Dietary Fiber	1 g	
1/2 Fat	**Total Fat**	4.5 g	**Potassium**	250 mg	Sugars	3 g	
	Saturated Fat	0.9 g			**Protein**	9 g	
	Trans Fat	0.0 g			**Phosphorus**	55 mg	

SUMMER TUNA SALAD WITH SALAD BAR VEGETABLES

Servings: 4 | Serving Size: 1 1/4 cups | Prep Time: 20 minutes | Cook Time: 0

Years ago, I tired of the usual mayonnaise-based tuna salad. I found it heavy and all that creamy dressing muddied the flavors. Here, I have created a clean-tasting tuna salad filled with fresh veggies and a light balsamic dressing to marry all the flavors beautifully.

1 cup	halved cherry or grape tomatoes (if cherry tomatoes are large, quarter them)
1 cup	sliced or shredded zucchini
1 cup	shredded or sliced carrots
1/2 cup	red bell pepper strips
1/4 cup	diced red onion
2 cups	flaked white meat tuna (canned in water and drained)

Dressing

3 tablespoons	balsamic vinegar
2 teaspoons	Dijon mustard
1	garlic clove, minced
1/2 teaspoon	dried basil
1/4 teaspoon	sugar
	pinch crushed red pepper flakes
3 Tbsp	olive oil
	dash sea salt
1/4 teaspoon	freshly ground black pepper

1. Combine the cherry tomatoes, zucchini, carrots, red pepper strips, and red onion in a large bowl. Fold in the tuna and mix well.

2. In a small bowl or measuring cup, whisk together the vinegar, mustard, garlic, basil, sugar, and crushed red pepper flakes. Slowly in a thin stream, whisk in the olive oil until emulsified. Season with salt and pepper. Add to the tuna salad and mix gently. Serve over greens, if desired.

Exchanges/Choices

2 Vegetable	**Calories**	290	**Cholesterol**	50 mg	**Total Carbohydrate**	10 g	
4 Lean Meat	Calories from Fat	125	**Sodium**	575 mg	Dietary Fiber	2 g	
1 1/2 Fat	**Total Fat**	14.0 g	**Potassium**	625 mg	Sugars	6 g	
	Saturated Fat	2.4 g			**Protein**	30 g	
	Trans Fat	0.0 g			**Phosphorus**	305 mg	

ROASTED CHERRY TOMATO
AND RED PEPPER PENNE

Servings: 4   Serving Size: 1 1/2 cups   Prep Time: 15 minutes   Cook Time: 20 minutes

This is really two recipes in one! Roasted cherry tomatoes and red peppers are simply divine on their own as a side dish. When combined with whole-wheat pasta and a dash of olives and capers, you'll have a family favorite to prepare over and over again.

2 cups	halved cherry tomatoes
2 cups	sliced red pepper strips
2	garlic cloves, finely minced
1 1/2 tablespoons	olive oil
1/4 teaspoon	Kosher salt
1/4 teaspoon	freshly ground black pepper
1 tablespoon	small capers, drained
1/4 cup	sliced pitted Kalamata olives
1/4 cup	sliced fresh basil
4 cups	hot cooked whole-wheat penne noodles

1 Preheat the oven to 425 degrees. Line 2 large baking sheets with parchment paper or non-stick foil.

2 Combine the cherry tomatoes, red pepper strips, garlic, oil, salt, and pepper and mix well. Arrange the tomatoes and red peppers in a single layer on the baking sheets. Roast the vegetables for about 20–25 minutes until tender.

3 Remove the vegetables from the oven and add them to a large bowl. Add in the capers, olives, and basil. Serve the vegetable sauce over the cooked penne noodles.

Exchanges/Choices

2 Starch	**Calories**	275	**Cholesterol**	0 mg	**Total Carbohydrate**	42 g
1 Vegetable	Calories from Fat	80	**Sodium**	330 mg	Dietary Fiber	7 g
2 Fat	**Total Fat**	9.0 g	**Potassium**	370 mg	Sugars	6 g
	Saturated Fat	1.1 g			**Protein**	7 g
	Trans Fat	0.0 g			**Phosphorus**	115 mg

CHAPTER 4

¼ lb. of this, ¼ lb. of that from the Deli Counter

I remember when the deli counter in the grocery store was small and tucked in the corner in an obscure part of the store. Today, the deli is a goldmine of foods, a plethora for you to use to assemble perfectly fine meals.

Many of the recipes in this section feature the fresh deli meats on display in most delis. The difference is that I incorporate them in new ways. Once thought of as just sandwich filling, you will find that adding deli meat to entrees makes it easy to prepare creative meals any day of the week.

My first suggestion is to find delis that roast their own meat in the store. Often beautifully displayed and definitely enticing, these are roasted just like you would do at home. Most store delis across the country offer really good brands of lower sodium meats, such as Boars Head, Dietz and Watson, and Wellshire Farms. Gone are the days where you might purchase what I call "meat surprise": slices of meat with so many chemicals, and with a rubbery texture that is unappealing and tasteless. You should have no trouble getting clean tasting, chemical free, lower sodium chicken, turkey, and beef at a store near you.

Make sure to check out the other offerings of today's deli. Store made hummus, tabouli salad, salsa, and roasted vegetable salads are all used in this chapter. Most stores are very good about having the ingredients listed for you and often include nutritional information. So, dig into *Stuffed Tomatoes with Tabouli* (pg 69), *Toasted Vegetable Baguette* (pg 70), or *Mexican Chicken* (pg 63) knowing that much of the work has been done and you can enjoy the delicious results courtesy of that "little" deli counter you'll no longer overlook!

PEA, TOMATO, AND HAM SALAD

This is a great salad for toting to picnics and all other summer fun activities—a refreshing change from leafy green salads. It will be in your summer cooking repertoire for a long time.

1 (16-ounce) package	frozen peas, thawed
1 1/3 cups	diced low-sodium deli ham
2 medium	tomatoes, diced
2	scallions, minced

Dressing

2 tablespoons	champagne vinegar
1 teaspoon	Dijon mustard
1	garlic clove, minced
1/2 teaspoon	sugar
3 tablespoons	olive oil
1/4 teaspoon	freshly ground black pepper

1. In a large bowl, mix together the peas, ham, tomatoes, and scallions.

2. In a small bowl, whisk together the vinegar, mustard, garlic, and sugar. Slowly in a thin stream, whisk in the olive oil until dressing is emulsified. Season with pepper. Pour the dressing over the pea salad and mix well.

3. Cover and refrigerate for 1 hour prior to serving.

Exchanges/Choices

1 Starch	**Calories**	265	**Cholesterol**	25 mg	**Total Carbohydrate**	22 g
2 Lean Meat	Calories from Fat	115	**Sodium**	585 mg	Dietary Fiber	6 g
2 Fat	**Total Fat**	13.0 g	**Potassium**	505 mg	Sugars	8 g
	Saturated Fat	2.3 g			**Protein**	16 g
	Trans Fat	0.0 g			**Phosphorus**	205 mg

MEXICAN CHICKEN

Servings: 4
Prep Time: 10 minutes

Serving Size: 4 ounces chicken, 6 ounces sauce
Cook Time: 40 minutes

While making your own salsa is fun, why not pick up some fresh salsa from the deli counter. Simply mix it with creamy fat-free sour cream and a kick of Southwestern spices, pour over chicken, and you have an easy weeknight meal.

1 1/2 cups	deli-fresh salsa
1 cup	fat-free sour cream
1/4 cup	minced fresh cilantro
1/4 cup	lower-fat shredded cheddar cheese (such as Cabot 50%)
2 teaspoons	salt-free Southwest seasoning, such as Mrs. Dash
1 pound	boneless skinless chicken breasts

1. Preheat the oven to 350 degrees. Coat a large baking dish with cooking spray. In a medium bowl, mix together the salsa, sour cream, cilantro, and cheese.

2. Sprinkle both sides of each chicken breast with the Southwest seasoning. Add the chicken breasts to the prepared pan. Pour the sauce over the chicken. Bake for about 40 minutes until the chicken registers 170 degrees on a meat thermometer.

Exchanges/Choices

1 Carbohydrate
4 Lean Meat

Calories	225	**Cholesterol**	75 mg	**Total Carbohydrate**	16 g
Calories from Fat	40	**Sodium**	475 mg	Dietary Fiber	2 g
Total Fat	4.5 g	**Potassium**	585 mg	Sugars	5 g
Saturated Fat	1.9 g			**Protein**	30 g
Trans Fat	0.0 g			**Phosphorus**	305 mg

DELI CHICKEN GYROS

Servings: 4　　　Serving Size: 1 sandwich　　　Prep Time: 15 minutes　　　Cook Time: 5 minutes

Every time I have traveled to Greece, I skip most of the more formal meals in favor of visiting a place with great gyros. But you don't have to travel to an ancient civilization to bring the Greek flavor to your table. These fresh-tasting sandwiches are a breeze to prepare as the deli has cooked chicken ready to use!

Sauce

1 cup	fat-free plain Greek yogurt, drained of any excess water
1/2 cup	peeled, seeded, diced cucumber
2 tablespoons	minced onion
1 teaspoon	minced garlic
4 (6-inch)	whole-wheat pita breads

Filling

4 ounces	diced cooked low-sodium chicken breasts
3/4 cup	seeded, diced tomatoes
1/2 cup	shredded lettuce
1/2 cup	minced scallions
2 tablespoons	feta cheese

1. Preheat the oven to 400 degrees. In a small bowl, combine the sauce ingredients.

2. Wrap the pita breads in foil. Add the pita bread to the oven and heat for about 5 minutes until warmed through.

3. For each serving, place the pita bread on a plate. Divide the filling ingredients and sauce among all pita breads. Fold the pita bread into a pocket. You may wrap the bottom of each gyro in foil before serving.

Exchanges/Choices

2 Starch	**Calories**	255	**Cholesterol**	20 mg	**Total Carbohydrate**	41 g	
1/2 Carbohydrate	Calories from Fat	25	**Sodium**	595 mg	Dietary Fiber	6 g	
2 Lean Meat	**Total Fat**	3.0 g	**Potassium**	415 mg	Sugars	5 g	
	Saturated Fat	1.0 g			**Protein**	19 g	
	Trans Fat	0.0 g			**Phosphorus**	290 mg	

ROAST BEEF ROLLUPS

Stuck for new ideas for lunch? Rollups are easy to pack in any lunch bag. Just pick up some beautifully roasted beef and tuck it inside layers of whole-wheat tortilla and vegetables. Eating a sandwich has never been easier or tasted so good.

6 (10-inch)	whole-wheat flour tortillas
6 large	romaine lettuce leaves
12 ounces	thinly sliced cooked deli roast beef
1 cup	diced tomatoes
1 cup	diced red bell pepper
1 tablespoon	olive oil
1 tablespoon	red wine vinegar
1 teaspoon	cumin
1/4 teaspoon	freshly ground black pepper

1. For each rollup, tear a 15-inch piece of either waxed paper or foil. Place the tortilla flat on the paper or foil. Place a romaine lettuce leaf on top of each tortilla. Divide the beef onto the lettuce leaves.

2. Combine the tomatoes, red peppers, oil, vinegar, cumin, and pepper. Divide the tomato mixture over the beef.

3. Roll the paper or foil over the tortilla to encase the filling. Roll until the sandwich is completely rolled up. Fold the excess paper or foil over the top and bottom of each rollup. To eat, peel back the paper or foil.

Exchanges/Choices

2 1/2 Starch
2 Lean Meat

Calories	295	**Cholesterol**	30 mg	**Total Carbohydrate**	43 g
Calories from Fat	55	**Sodium**	595 mg	Dietary Fiber	6 g
Total Fat	6.0 g	**Potassium**	480 mg	Sugars	3 g
Saturated Fat	1.6 g			**Protein**	19 g
Trans Fat	0.0 g			**Phosphorus**	270 mg

QUICK HOPPIN' JOHN

Servings: 6   **Serving Size:** 1 cup   **Prep Time:** 20 minutes   **Cook Time:** 35 minutes

When I was in graduate school, one of the women I lived with made Hoppin' John all the time. Not being from the southern United States, I was intrigued by the combination of black-eyed peas, collard greens, and turkey. While traditional Hoppin' John takes longer to prepare, this recipe utilizes a few shortcuts and remains the perfect comfort food that your friends and family will enjoy anytime.

1 tablespoon	canola oil
1 medium	onion, chopped
1/2 cup	diced carrots
1/2 cup	diced celery
2	garlic cloves, minced
1 cup	long-grain brown rice
2 cups	low-fat, low-sodium chicken broth
2 (15-ounce) cans	black-eyed peas
1 (10-ounce) package	frozen collard greens, slightly thawed
1 teaspoon	fresh minced thyme
1 cup	diced low-sodium deli turkey breast
1/4 teaspoon	Kosher salt
1/4 teaspoon	freshly ground black pepper

1. Heat the oil in a large skillet over medium heat. Add the onions, carrots, and celery and sauté for 6–7 minutes. Add in the garlic and sauté for 2 minutes. Add in the rice and sauté for 2 minutes.

2. Add in the broth, bring to a boil, cover, and simmer on low heat for about 35–40 minutes. In the last 10 minutes of the rice cooking, add the peas, collard greens, and thyme, cover, and continue to simmer until rice is tender.

3. Add in the turkey, salt, and pepper and gently mix and cook for 2 minutes.

Exchanges/Choices

2 1/2 Starch	**Calories**	315	**Cholesterol**	15 mg	**Total Carbohydrate**	52 g
2 Vegetable	Calories from Fat	40	**Sodium**	465 mg	Dietary Fiber	10 g
1 Lean Meat	**Total Fat**	4.5 g	**Potassium**	665 mg	Sugars	6 g
1/2 Fat	Saturated Fat	0.6 g			**Protein**	18 g
	Trans Fat	0.0 g			**Phosphorus**	340 mg

TURKEY AND CRANBERRY SALAD

Servings: 4   Serving Size: 1 1/4 cups   Prep Time: 20 minutes   Cook Time: 0

This pretty jewel-colored salad is perfect for the holidays. Why not serve it for a festive brunch along with some fresh whole-grain rolls and a side of steamed French green beans.

2 cups	diced cooked low-sodium deli turkey breast
1/2 cup	dried unsweetened cranberries
1/2 cup	diced red bell pepper
1/2 cup	diced yellow bell pepper
1/4 cup	diced red onion
2 tablespoons	minced scallions

Dressing

2 tablespoons	raspberry vinegar
1 teaspoon	Dijon mustard
1/2 teaspoon	sugar
3 tablespoons	olive oil
	pinch sea salt
1/4 teaspoon	freshly ground black pepper

1 In a large bowl, combine the turkey, cranberries, red and yellow peppers, red onion, and scallions.

2 In a small bowl, whisk together the vinegar, mustard, and sugar. Slowly, in a thin stream, whisk in the olive oil until the dressing is emulsified. Season with salt and pepper. Pour the dressing over the salad and gently mix.

Exchanges/Choices

1 Carbohydrate	**Calories**	205	**Cholesterol**	30 mg	**Total Carbohydrate**	12 g
2 Lean Meat	Calories from Fat	100	**Sodium**	445 mg	Dietary Fiber	3 g
1 1/2 Fat	**Total Fat**	11.0 g	**Potassium**	320 mg	Sugars	6 g
	Saturated Fat	1.7 g			**Protein**	16 g
	Trans Fat	0.0 g			**Phosphorus**	175 mg

BARBEQUED ROAST BEEF OPEN-FACED SANDWICHES

Servings: 4   Serving Size: 1 sandwich   Prep Time: 10 minutes   marinating time: 1 hour

Deli roast beef gets a little upgrade by marinating it in zesty spices. Why settle for a plain roast beef sandwich when you can jazz it up with these delicious sandwiches?

Marinade

1/3 cup	fresh lemon juice
2 tablespoons	olive oil
3 tablespoons	minced onion
1 tablespoon	mild or hot chili powder
2 teaspoons	paprika
1/4 teaspoon	ground cumin
1/4 teaspoon	ground ginger
12 ounces	sliced cooked deli roast beef
4 slices	whole-wheat or rye bread
8 slices	tomato

1. In a bowl, mix together the marinade ingredients. Pour the marinade into a shallow baking pan. Add the roast beef slices and turn to coat. Cover and marinate in the refrigerator for 1 hour.

2. Remove the roast beef from the refrigerator and allow it to come to room temperature, about 15 minutes. Drain any excess marinade from the roast beef.

3. Toast the bread slices. Divide the roast beef among all the bread slices. Top with 2 tomato slices per sandwich.

Exchanges/Choices

1 Starch	**Calories**	255	**Cholesterol**	50 mg	**Total Carbohydrate**	21 g
3 Lean Meat	Calories from Fat	90	**Sodium**	530 mg	Dietary Fiber	7 g
1 Fat	**Total Fat**	10.0 g	**Potassium**	655 mg	Sugars	5 g
	Saturated Fat	2.5 g			**Protein**	23 g
	Trans Fat	0.0 g			**Phosphorus**	260 mg

STUFFED TOMATOES WITH TABOULI

Servings: 4   Serving Size: 1 tomato   Prep Time: 20 minutes   Standing time: 1 hour

Who has time to prepare tabouli salad from scratch? Fortunately, many delis offer prepared tabouli, which makes it perfect to fix this Middle Eastern inspired stuffed tomato. A dollop of creamy hummus puts the finishing touch on this perfect summer luncheon entree.

1 cup	tabouli salad from deli
1 cup	peeled, seeded, and diced cucumber
1 cup	diced cooked deli chicken breast
4 medium	ripe, firm tomatoes
2 teaspoons	olive oil
4 tablespoons	hummus from deli

1. In a bowl, combine the tabouli salad, cucumber, and chicken and mix well. Cover and refrigerate for 1 hour.

2. Cut off the top of each tomato with a small paring knife. With a grapefruit spoon, carefully scoop out the tomato pulp, removing the seeds from each tomato.

3. Divide the tabouli mixture among all the tomatoes. Drizzle each tomato with olive oil and top with a dollop of hummus.

Exchanges/Choices

1/2 Starch	**Calories**	150	**Cholesterol**	10 mg	**Total Carbohydrate**	16 g
1 Vegetable	Calories from Fat	45	**Sodium**	445 mg	Dietary Fiber	4 g
1 Lean Meat	**Total Fat**	5.0 g	**Potassium**	490 mg	Sugars	6 g
1 Fat	Saturated Fat	0.8 g			**Protein**	11 g
	Trans Fat	0.0 g			**Phosphorus**	160 mg

TOASTED VEGETABLE BAGUETTE

Servings: 4 | **Serving Size:** 1 sandwich | **Prep Time:** 15 minutes | **Cook Time:** 5 minutes

Vegetable sandwiches, while they sound healthy, can be anything but. Usually drowning in oil and too much cheese, these lightened up sandwiches are perfect when you want to take a rest from meat. And the carb count goes down by eliminating some of the unnecessary bread filling.

4 (6-inch)	mini baguettes, split in half the long way
1 pound	roasted vegetable salad from the deli, drained of the oil
1/4 cup	minced parsley
2 ounces	shredded reduced-fat cheddar cheese

1 Preheat the oven to 350 degrees. For each baguette, remove most of the bread to create a hollow shell for both pieces.

2 Fill the one side of shell with the vegetable salad. Sprinkle with parsley and top with cheddar cheese. Close the sandwich.

3 Place the sandwiches on a baking sheet and bake for 5 minutes until cheese melts.

Exchanges/Choices

1 Starch	**Calories**	185	**Cholesterol**	5 mg	**Total Carbohydrate**	23 g
2 Vegetable	Calories from Fat	70	**Sodium**	245 mg	Dietary Fiber	3 g
1 1/2 Fat	**Total Fat**	8.0 g	**Potassium**	365 mg	Sugars	6 g
	Saturated Fat	2.5 g			**Protein**	8 g
	Trans Fat	0.0 g			**Phosphorus**	145 mg

BARBEQUED CHICKEN SANDWICHES

Servings: 4   **Serving Size:** 1 sandwich   **Prep Time:** 10 minutes   **Cook Time:** 20 minutes

Rotisserie chickens are a great deli staple for your refrigerator. Here, we shred the breast meat and smother it in a homemade barbeque sauce. Keep cooked rotisserie chickens on hand for tacos and enchiladas, salads, soups, and stews.

Sauce

2/3 cup	low-sodium ketchup
1/2 cup	apple cider vinegar
2 teaspoons	fresh lemon juice
2 teaspoons	Worcestershire sauce
2 teaspoons	brown sugar
2 teaspoons	chili powder
1 teaspoon	paprika
1 teaspoon	cumin
1/4 teaspoon	cayenne pepper
1/4 teaspoon	freshly ground black pepper
2 cups	shredded rotisserie chicken, skinned and boned (use the white meat only)
4	whole-wheat buns, split and toasted

1. In a medium saucepan, combine all the ingredients for the sauce. Bring to a boil, lower the heat, and simmer uncovered, stirring occasionally, until the sauce thickens for about 15 minutes.

2. Add the chicken and cook for 5 minutes. Remove from the heat.

3. Spoon the chicken mixture on the bottom side of the bun. Top each with the other half of the bun.

Exchanges/Choices

2 Starch	**Calories**	295	**Cholesterol**	60 mg	**Total Carbohydrate**	40 g
1/2 Carbohydrate	Calories from Fat	45	**Sodium**	465 mg	Dietary Fiber	4 g
3 Lean Meat	**Total Fat**	5.0 g	**Potassium**	615 mg	Sugars	17 g
	Saturated Fat	1.0 g			**Protein**	25 g
	Trans Fat	0.0 g			**Phosphorus**	305 mg

FRUITY CHICKEN SALAD

Servings: 4	Serving Size: 1 cup	Prep Time: 15 minutes	Cook Time: 0

I first had fruit and chicken together when I visited the Caribbean as a young teen. It was such a treat to be greeted by a fresh pineapple stuffed with a mound of fresh chicken salad studded with ripe juicy fruit. Here, I've streamlined the presentation sans the pineapple shell, but I think you will feel transported to the islands after just one bite of this delectable salad.

2 cups	diced cooked fresh deli chicken
1/2 cup	diced red bell pepper (from salad bar)
1/2 cup	diced fresh pineapple (from salad bar or produce section)
1/2 cup	halved red grapes (from salad bar or produce section)
1/2 cup	diced cantaloupe (from salad bar or produce section)
1/4 cup	diced red onion

Dressing

1/2 cup	plain nonfat yogurt
1/2 cup	fat-free mayonnaise
2 tablespoons	fat-free sour cream
3 tablespoons	fresh orange juice
1 tablespoon	honey
1/2 teaspoon	fresh orange zest

1 In a large bowl, combine the chicken, red peppers, pineapple, grapes, cantaloupe, and red onion.

2 In a small bowl, whisk together the dressing ingredients. Pour over the salad and refrigerate until serving time.

Exchanges/Choices

1/2 Fruit	**Calories**	220	**Cholesterol**	85 mg	**Total Carbohydrate**	23 g	
1 Carbohydrate	Calories from Fat	55	**Sodium**	545 mg	Dietary Fiber	2 g	
3 Lean Meat	**Total Fat**	6.0 g	**Potassium**	490 mg	Sugars	17 g	
	Saturated Fat	1.4 g			**Protein**	22 g	
	Trans Fat	0.1 g			**Phosphorus**	255 mg	

ROASTED CHICKEN SALAD

Servings: 4   Serving Size: 1 cup   Prep Time: 10 minutes   Cook Time: 8 minutes

In the 80's, it was a restaurant trend to serve Asian-style chicken salad. Order up some fresh cooked deli chicken and toss with crunchy vegetables. Then, bathe it all in a tangy Asian dressing and you've got a tradition worth keeping.

1 teaspoon	toasted sesame oil
1 cup	thinly sliced carrots (from salad bar or produce section)
2	garlic cloves, minced
1 cup	fresh snow peas, halved
12 ounces	roasted deli chicken, cubed or shredded
1/2 cup	low-fat Oriental-style salad dressing or balsamic vinaigrette
2 cups	shredded Napa cabbage
1/4 cup	toasted cashews

1 Heat the oil in a large skillet over medium heat. Add the carrots and sauté for 3 minutes. Add the garlic and sauté for 1 minute. Add the snow peas, cover, and cook for 2 minutes. Add in the chicken and sauté for 2 minutes. Add in the dressing and remove from the heat.

2 Add the cabbage to a large bowl. Add in the chicken mixture and toss gently. Add the salad to individual plates and top with cashews.

Exchanges/Choices

1/2 Carbohydrate	**Calories**	265	**Cholesterol**	95 mg	**Total Carbohydrate**	15 g
1 Vegetable	Calories from Fat	100	**Sodium**	365 mg	Dietary Fiber	3 g
3 Lean Meat	**Total Fat**	11.0 g	**Potassium**	620 mg	Sugars	9 g
1 1/2 Fat	Saturated Fat	2.4 g			**Protein**	27 g
	Trans Fat	0.1 g			**Phosphorus**	305 mg

ITALIAN TURKEY SAUTE

Deli turkey goes far beyond its place between two slices of bread in this fantastic quick-skillet meal. Ask for a small amount of intensely flavored prosciutto at the deli along with the turkey. Add a few shelf-stable items such as capers and olives and you have a fast weekday Italian-style meal.

2 teaspoons	olive oil
1/4 cup	diced deli prosciutto
1/2 cup	diced onion
2	garlic cloves, finely minced
1 1/2 cups	crushed tomatoes
2 tablespoons	dry red wine
12 ounces	cubed low-sodium deli white meat turkey
2 tablespoons	minced fresh basil
2 teaspoons	capers
10	black pitted olives, halved

1. Heat the oil in a large skillet over medium heat. Add the prosciutto and sauté for 2 minutes. Add the onion and garlic and sauté for 4 minutes.

2. Add the tomatoes and red wine and bring to a boil. Lower the heat and simmer for 15 minutes.

3. Add in the turkey, basil, capers, and olives and cook for 2–3 minutes. Serve over rice or cooked pasta, if desired.

Exchanges/Choices

2 Vegetable
3 Lean Meat

Calories	185	**Cholesterol**	60 mg	**Total Carbohydrate**	10 g
Calories from Fat	45	**Sodium**	380 mg	Dietary Fiber	2 g
Total Fat	5.0 g	**Potassium**	615 mg	Sugars	5 g
Saturated Fat	0.8 g			**Protein**	26 g
Trans Fat	0.0 g			**Phosphorus**	240 mg

CHICKEN CORN SKILLET

Servings: 4
Prep Time: 15 minutes

Serving Size: 3 ounces chicken, 1/2 cup vegetables
Cook Time: 15 minutes

Skillet suppers are the most efficient way to get your vegetables and protein in just one pot. Toss fresh deli roasted chicken with some fresh vegetables from the salad bar and add convenient frozen corn to the mix and you've got dinner in about a half hour.

1 tablespoon	olive oil
12 ounces	deli roasted chicken, cut into 1-inch cubes
1 medium	onion, diced
1 medium	yellow squash, diced
1 medium	red bell pepper, diced
1/2 teaspoon	ground cumin
1/4 teaspoon	Kosher salt
1/4 teaspoon	freshly ground black pepper
2 cups	frozen corn, thawed
2 tablespoons	minced parsley

1. Heat the oil in a large skillet over medium-high heat. Add the chicken cubes and sauté for 2 minutes. Remove the chicken from the skillet and set aside.

2. Add the onion and sauté for 5 minutes. Add the squash and red pepper and sauté for 4 minutes. Add the cumin, salt, and pepper and sauté for 1 minute.

3. Add in the corn and parsley and sauté for 2 minutes. Add back the chicken and heat through for 1 minute.

Exchanges/Choices

1 Starch	**Calories**	260	**Cholesterol**	95 mg	**Total Carbohydrate**	21 g	
1 Vegetable	Calories from Fat	90	**Sodium**	455 mg	Dietary Fiber	4 g	
3 Lean Meat	**Total Fat**	10.0 g	**Potassium**	680 mg	Sugars	6 g	
1/2 Fat	Saturated Fat	2.0 g			**Protein**	27 g	
	Trans Fat	0.1 g			**Phosphorus**	305 mg	

CHICKEN AND ALMOND STEW

Servings: 4   Serving Size: 1 cup   Prep Time: 20 minutes   Cook Time: 45 minutes

Beef stew is always a welcomed dish, but how about something a bit different than the usual standby? Here, I've combined readymade cooked chicken with zesty ground spices, healthy black beans, and some crunchy toasted almonds to create a warming stew perfect for those autumn nights.

1 tablespoon	olive oil
1 medium	onion, chopped
2	garlic cloves, minced
1 teaspoon	mild chili powder
1/4 teaspoon	ground cinnamon
1/4 teaspoon	cayenne pepper
2 cups	fat-free, low-sodium chicken broth
1 cup	diced no-salt-added tomatoes, drained
1/4 cup	toasted slivered almonds
10 ounces	low-sodium deli roasted chicken, cut into 1-inch cubes
1 (15-ounce) can	black beans, rinsed and drained

1 Heat the oil in a large saucepot over medium heat. Add the onion and sauté for 5 minutes. Add the garlic, chili powder, cinnamon, and cayenne pepper, and sauté for 2 minutes.

2 Add in the broth and tomatoes and bring to a boil. Lower the heat and simmer on low for 30 minutes.

3 Add in the almonds, chicken, and black beans. Simmer for an additional 10 minutes.

Exchanges/Choices

1 Starch	**Calories**	255	**Cholesterol**	40 mg	**Total Carbohydrate**	23 g
1 Vegetable	Calories from Fat	70	**Sodium**	590 mg	Dietary Fiber	8 g
3 Lean Meat	**Total Fat**	8.0 g	**Potassium**	765 mg	Sugars	5 g
1/2 Fat	Saturated Fat	1.1 g			**Protein**	24 g
	Trans Fat	0.0 g			**Phosphorus**	320 mg

MEDITERRANEAN CHICKEN AND PASTA

Servings: 4
Prep Time: 20 minutes
Serving Size: 1/2 cup pasta, 1 1/2 ounces chicken, 3/4 cup spinach
Cook Time: 10–12 minutes

Be transported to a sunny Mediterranean island with a bowlful of this pretty pasta dish. The fresh kick of lemon zest and intense flavor of oregano and basil really perks up plain pasta. A nice light sprinkling of tangy feta cheese crowns this crowd pleaser.

1 tablespoon	olive oil
1 medium	onion, chopped
2	garlic cloves, minced
6 ounces	deli cooked chicken breasts, cut into 1/2-inch cubes
1 teaspoon	dried oregano
1 teaspoon	dried basil
1/4 teaspoon	crushed red pepper flakes
1/4 teaspoon	freshly ground black pepper
1/2 cup	low-fat, reduced-sodium chicken broth
1 teaspoon	grated lemon zest
3 cups	coarsely chopped fresh spinach (salad bar or produce section)
2 cups	cooked whole-wheat shells (or other shaped pasta)
1/4 cup	crumbled feta cheese

1. Heat the oil in a large skillet over medium heat. Add the onion and sauté for 5–6 minutes. Add in the garlic and sauté for 1 minute.

2. Add in the chicken, oregano, basil, crushed red pepper, and freshly ground black pepper and sauté for 2 minutes.

3. Pour in the broth and bring to a boil. Reduce the heat to low and add the lemon zest. Add in the spinach and cook just until spinach begins to wilt.

4. Add in the cooked pasta and toss very gently. Top each serving with feta cheese.

Exchanges/Choices

1 1/2 Starch	**Calories**	205	**Cholesterol**	25 mg	**Total Carbohydrate**	25 g
1 Vegetable	Calories from Fat	55	**Sodium**	545 mg	Dietary Fiber	3 g
1 Lean Meat	**Total Fat**	6.0 g	**Potassium**	360 mg	Sugars	4 g
1/2 Fat	Saturated Fat	2.1 g			**Protein**	15 g
	Trans Fat	0.1 g			**Phosphorus**	220 mg

SUN-DRIED TOMATO TURKEY SALAD

Servings: 4   Serving Size: about 1 cup   Prep Time: 20 minutes   Cook Time: 0

Sun-dried tomatoes can make any dish just taste better. I spare no flavor expense in my liberal use of the juicy sun-touched tomato in this lunch salad. Try this with deli chicken or roast beef as well.

12 ounces	no salt added deli turkey breast, cut into 1/2-inch cubes
1/2 cup	rehydrated sun-dried tomatoes, thinly sliced (not packed in oil)
1 large	carrot, peeled and diced
1	celery stalk, diced
1 medium	red bell pepper, cored, seeded, and diced
3	scallions, thinly sliced
1/4 cup	diced red onion

Dressing

1/2 cup	fat-free mayonnaise
1/4 cup	plain nonfat yogurt
1/4 cup	fat-free sour cream
1 tablespoon	prepared pesto
1/2 teaspoon	fresh lemon zest
1/4 teaspoon	Kosher salt
1/4 teaspoon	freshly ground black pepper
	Romaine lettuce leaves (optional)

1. In a large salad bowl, combine the turkey, sun-dried tomatoes, carrot, celery, red pepper, scallions, and red onion.

2. In a small bowl, whisk together the dressing ingredients. Add the dressing to the turkey salad and gently mix. Cover and refrigerate for 1/2 hour prior to serving. Serve over lettuce leaves if desired.

Exchanges/Choices

1/2 Carbohydrate	**Calories**	210	**Cholesterol**	60 mg	
2 Vegetable	Calories from Fat	30	**Sodium**	580 mg	
3 Lean Meat	**Total Fat**	3.5 g	**Potassium**	780 mg	
	Saturated Fat	0.8 g			
	Trans Fat	0.0 g			

Total Carbohydrate	19 g
Dietary Fiber	3 g
Sugars	11 g
Protein	26 g
Phosphorus	300 mg

CHAPTER 5

Freezer Short Cuts

I f all you want for dinner is an already prepared meal, you might spend time perusing the freezer section of the grocery for an appealing photo on the box of a TV dinner. While you certainly have your choice of hundreds of these, the fact is that the frozen food aisle offers so much more than already prepared, overly processed meals. The frozen aisle of your grocery or market can play an essential part in the preparation of quick and healthy homemade meals.

In this chapter, I offer ways to incorporate frozen vegetables and fruits that go well beyond being relegated to the side of the plate as an afterthought. The beauty of using frozen vegetables and fruits is that you can plan your meals ahead, without fear of spoilage. While eating fresh vegetables and fruits is always great, nutritionally speaking, frozen produce can be just as good as and sometimes even better than, fresh. After vegetables and fruits are picked, many are flash frozen and then shipped to grocery stores. Careful consideration is paid to make sure the produce is packaged quickly, which reduces exposure to light and air, two factors that decrease the nutritional content of food. There is also cost consideration. Often you will find that frozen fruits and vegetables are less expensive, and by purchasing them in bulk, you may actually save money and reduce your grocery shopping trips.

Frozen shrimp and chicken should be home freezer staples. I barely notice the difference in taste between these foods in their frozen state and when offered as fresh. While your supermarket almost always has these stocked in their freezer, if you have a warehouse-style store in your neighborhood, frozen shrimp and chicken are sold in larger amounts, often at considerable savings. Remember to use frozen proteins within 3 months for best results. Never leave a frozen product to thaw at room temperature. Leave a reminder for yourself to tuck it in the refrigerator to thaw overnight prior to use. Place the bag of frozen chicken or shrimp in a deep bowl or rimmed plate in the refrigerator so that juices to do not spill out onto your refrigerator shelves.

Take another look around your store's freezer and you just might find some other products that you can incorporate into your daily food plan. One such product is frozen brown rice. While cooking brown rice is not hard, frozen makes eating healthier a cinch for all of us. Usually packaged in a Ziploc bag, you can simply take out what you need and zip up the rest for another time. Frozen edamame is another great product to toss in your cart. Rich in protein and fiber, edamame makes a fabulous base for vegetarian main meals. All you need to do is open the bag, cook for a few minutes, and you have a healthy addition to the dinner table. Also check out your market's variety of frozen pastas. Depending on your store, I've seen many markets offer locally produced pastas, even whole-grain pasta, to give a local producer a chance to display their creations. These are often quite tasty and you'll be supporting the local movement.

A few tips for home storage and use of frozen foods:

1. Shop in the freezer department of the market as your last stop before you check-out. Although most products are solidly frozen, all it takes is a short amount of time out of the freezer for products to begin thawing. If you need to purchase quite a bit, consider toting along a small portable insulated container so products stay frozen for the trip home. And with lots of frozen foods in the car, go directly home.

2. Don't overstuff your freezer. While closely positioned items are fine, don't cram the freezer beyond its capacity. You'll lose track of what you have and foods may begin to stick to each other.

3. If you need to rewrap foods be sure to completely cover the food item to prevent freezer burn. Best to wrap in butcher paper first, followed by slipping it into a heavy Ziploc freezer bag.

4. Label and date everything you place in the freezer.

5. For more storage efficiency, stack your frozen foods on top of each other. Avoid placing awkwardly shaped containers of different sizes onto the freezer shelves. Try to stack neatly.

6. Make it a habit to clean out your freezer regularly. I'm sure there will be products you have decided you don't want to eat or have gone beyond their expiration time. Check frequently to cut down waste.

SHRIMP AND BELL PEPPER TACOS

Servings: 6   Serving Size: 1 taco   Prep Time: 20 minutes   Cook Time: 13 minutes

I love perusing the frozen veggie section of the market; there is something different everyday in the freezer section, or so it seems. One of my favorite products to use is the bell pepper medleys, which bulk up this taco in a most nutritious, yet flavorful way.

6 ounces	frozen large shrimp, peeled and deveined, thawed, and patted dry
1/2 teaspoon	ground cumin
1/2 teaspoon	dried oregano leaves
1/4 teaspoon	ground black pepper
1/8 teaspoon	cayenne pepper
1 tablespoon	vegetable oil, divided
1 (16-ounce) bag	frozen pepper medley
3	garlic cloves, minced
1 tablespoon	fresh lime juice
6 (8-inch)	whole-wheat flour tortillas
6 tablespoons	shredded reduced-fat cheddar cheese
1/2 cup	fat-free sour cream or plain Greek yogurt, stirred

1 In a medium bowl, combine the thawed shrimp with the cumin, oregano, salt, black pepper, and cayenne.

2 Heat 2 teaspoons of the oil in a large heavy skillet over medium-high heat. Add the shrimp and sauté for about 2–3 minutes or until shrimp is cooked through. Remove the shrimp with a slotted spoon.

3 Add remaining oil to the skillet and add the pepper medley. Sauté the peppers for about 5 minutes. Add the garlic and sauté for about 2 minutes. Drain off any excess liquid. Add the lime juice and cook for 30 seconds. Add back the cooked shrimp and toss to coat with the peppers.

4 Heat the whole-wheat tortillas by toasting them one at a time in a medium skillet over medium heat for about 1–2 minutes per side.

5 Divide the shrimp-pepper mixture between all six tortillas. Fold over, sprinkle with cheese, and top with sour cream or yogurt.

Exchanges/Choices

2 Starch	**Calories**	250	**Cholesterol**	50 mg	**Total Carbohydrate**	38 g
1 Vegetable	Calories from Fat	45	**Sodium**	585 mg	Dietary Fiber	5 g
1 Lean Meat	**Total Fat**	5.0 g	**Potassium**	300 mg	Sugars	4 g
1/2 Fat	Saturated Fat	1.4 g			**Protein**	15 g
	Trans Fat	0.0 g			**Phosphorus**	250 mg

TORTELLINI WITH SHRIMP AND SPINACH

Servings: 5 | Serving Size: 1 cup | Prep Time: 10 minutes | Cook Time: 25 minutes

Refrigerated or frozen pastas are such a great staple to have on hand. With the help of frozen spinach and shelf-stable canned tomatoes, this one-pot dish tastes rich with the addition of some creamy texture provided by fat-free half and half. This is the perfect dish for a seasonably cool autumn evening.

1 (9-ounce) package	reduced-fat cheese tortellini (such as Buitoni)
1 tablespoon	olive oil
1/2 cup	minced onion
3	garlic cloves, minced
1 (10-ounce) package	frozen chopped spinach, partially thawed
1 (14.5-ounce) can	no-salt-added diced tomatoes with Italian herbs, drained
1/4 teaspoon	freshly ground black pepper
8 ounces	cooked large peeled and deveined shrimp, thawed and patted dry
1/4 cup	fat-free half and half
	pinch crushed red pepper flakes
1/4 cup	fresh sliced basil

1. Prepare the tortellini according to package directions.

2. Meanwhile, heat the olive oil in a large skillet over medium heat. Add the onion and garlic and sauté for 3–4 minutes. Add in the spinach, breaking it up with a wooden spoon. Cook the spinach for 3–4 minutes. Drain off any excess liquid. Drain the tortellini and set aside.

3. Add the tomatoes and pepper to the spinach and reduce the heat to low and simmer for 3 minutes. Add in the cooked shrimp and tortellini and cook 1 minute.

4. Stir in the half and half and the red pepper flakes. Cook for 2 minutes. Garnish with fresh basil.

Exchanges/Choices

1 1/2 Starch	**Calories**	260	**Cholesterol**	80 mg	**Total Carbohydrate**	32 g
1 Vegetable	Calories from Fat	70	**Sodium**	580 mg	Dietary Fiber	5 g
2 Lean Meat	**Total Fat**	8.0 g	**Potassium**	450 mg	Sugars	5 g
1/2 Fat	Saturated Fat	2.1 g			**Protein**	17 g
	Trans Fat	0.0 g			**Phosphorus**	260 mg

CHICKEN IN BLUEBERRY SAUCE

Servings: 4   Serving Size: 4 ounce chicken breast   Prep Time: 5 minutes Cook Time: 25 minutes

Get your dessert in your main dish! Frozen blueberries are for so much more than eating out of hand or adding to the usual smoothie. Making this jewel-colored sauce dotted with wild blueberries elevates chicken to definite new heights.

4 (4-ounce)	chicken breasts fresh or frozen, thawed and patted dry
1/2 teaspoon	Kosher salt
1/4 teaspoon	freshly ground black pepper
1 tablespoon	olive oil
1/2 cup	no-sugar-added apricot preserves
2 tablespoons	Dijon mustard
1/3 cup	cider vinegar
3/4 cup	frozen wild blueberries, thawed and drained

1 Sprinkle the chicken with salt and pepper. Heat the oil in a large skillet over medium-high heat.

2 Sear the chicken on both sides for about 5–6 minutes per side. Combine the preserves and mustard and pour over the chicken. Cover the chicken and simmer on low heat for about 10–15 minutes.

3 Remove the chicken with a slotted spoon and keep warm. Add the vinegar to the pan and bring to a boil. Lower the heat and simmer for 3–4 minutes until the sauce is reduced by one third. Add in the blueberries. Taste and correct for seasoning. Serve the sauce over the chicken.

Exchanges/Choices

1 Carbohydrate	**Calories**	205	**Cholesterol**	65 mg	**Total Carbohydrate**	15 g
3 Lean Meat	Calories from Fat	65	**Sodium**	480 mg	Dietary Fiber	1 g
	Total Fat	7.0 g	**Potassium**	270 mg	Sugars	3 g
	Saturated Fat	1.3 g			**Protein**	24 g
	Trans Fat	0.0 g			**Phosphorus**	190 mg

HASH BROWN QUICHE

I could never master making a flour crust for quiches. So, when I found a shredded frozen hash browns, I took advantage! The crust is hearty and filling while the filling is light and fluffy. Use this crust idea and fill it with your favorite quiche flavors.

2 teaspoons	olive oil
1 medium	onion, chopped
2	garlic cloves, minced
1 (10-ounce) package	chopped frozen spinach, slightly thawed
1/4 teaspoon	nutmeg
1/2 teaspoon	Kosher salt
1/4 teaspoon	freshly ground black pepper
1/4 teaspoon	hot sauce
1 1/2 cups	frozen hash browns (such as Ore-Ida), thawed and drained and patted dry
2	whole eggs
4	egg whites
1/2 cup	1% milk
1/3 cup	reduced-fat shredded cheddar cheese
2 tablespoons	grated fresh Parmesan cheese

1. Preheat the oven to 350 degrees. Heat the oil in a large skillet over medium heat. Add the onion and garlic and sauté for 5 minutes. Add in the spinach, breaking it up until spinach is completely thawed and cooked. Drain any excess water. Add in the nutmeg, salt, pepper, and hot sauce.

2. Coat a 9-inch pie or quiche pan with cooking spray. Add the spinach to the bottom of the pie pan, spreading it evenly across the bottom. Add a layer of the hash browns on top of the spinach.

3. Whisk together the eggs, egg whites, milk, and cheeses. Pour the egg-milk mixture over the hash browns. Bake the quiche for about 25–30 minutes until the top is set.

Exchanges/Choices

1/2 Carbohydrate	**Calories**	90	**Cholesterol**	50 mg	**Total Carbohydrate**	8 g
1 Lean Meat	Calories from Fat	35	**Sodium**	260 mg	Dietary Fiber	2 g
1/2 Fat	**Total Fat**	4.0 g	**Potassium**	245 mg	Sugars	2 g
	Saturated Fat	1.5 g			**Protein**	7 g
	Trans Fat	0.0 g			**Phosphorus**	105 mg

CHICKEN WITH PEACH GINGER SAUCE

Servings: 4   Serving Size: 4 ounces   Prep Time: 10 minutes   Cook Time: 35 minutes

Get twice the flavor when you combine two peach flavors into one dish! This easy-to-do everyday dish benefits from a double dose of the fuzzy fruit in peach preserves and frozen peach slices. Delicious over boneless chicken breasts as I show it here, and try it over seared pork medallions as well!

1 1/2 tablespoons	olive oil, divided
1 tablespoon	fresh peeled and grated ginger
1	garlic clove, minced
1 cup	no-sugar-added peach preserves
1 cup	water
3 tablespoons	cider vinegar
2 cups	frozen peach slices
2 tablespoons	all purpose flour
1/2 teaspoon	Kosher salt
1/2 teaspoon	ground cumin
1/4 teaspoon	ground coriander
1/4 teaspoon	freshly ground black pepper
2	egg whites, beaten
4 (4-ounce)	boneless, skinless fresh or frozen chicken breasts, thawed, and patted dry

1 Heat 2 teaspoons of olive oil in a large saucepan over medium heat. Add in the ginger and garlic and sauté for 1 minute. Add in the peach preserves, water, and cider vinegar and cook for 4 minutes. Add in the peach slices, lower the heat, and simmer for 20 minutes until sauce is thick.

2 Meanwhile, on a plate, mix together the flour, salt, cumin, coriander, and ground black pepper. Dip the chicken in the egg whites and then coat each side of the chicken in the flour mixture.

3 Heat the remaining olive oil in a nonstick large skillet over medium-high heat. Add the chicken breasts and sear on both sides for about 6–7 minutes per side. Serve the chicken with the sauce.

Exchanges/Choices

2 Carbohydrate	**Calories**	275	**Cholesterol**	65 mg	**Total Carbohydrate**	32 g
3 Lean Meat	Calories from Fat	70	**Sodium**	325 mg	Dietary Fiber	9 g
	Total Fat	8.0 g	**Potassium**	475 mg	Sugars	8 g
	Saturated Fat	1.5 g			**Protein**	27 g
	Trans Fat	0.0 g			**Phosphorus**	205 mg

CLASSIC SPINACH PIE

Servings: 24   **Serving Size:** 2 × 2 inch square   **Prep Time:** 25 minutes   **Cook Time:** 36 minutes

One of my fondest memories is my mom, sister, and I preparing spinach pie every Sunday. Back then, we didn't hesitate to add loads of butter, but now we know that's not necessary, as cooking spray does the trick. The freezer section provides the most important ingredients; all you need to do is add some love.

	olive oil flavored cooking spray
2 teaspoons	olive oil
1 large	onion, chopped
2	garlic cloves, minced
3 (16-ounce) packages	frozen chopped spinach, thawed, drained, and squeezed dry
3/4 cup	crumbled feta cheese
2	eggs, beaten
1/4 teaspoon	Kosher salt
1/4 teaspoon	freshly ground black pepper
1 (1-pound) box	frozen filo dough, thawed according to package directions

1. Preheat the oven to 400 degrees. Coat a 9 × 13-inch baking dish with cooking spray. Set aside. Heat the oil in a medium skillet over medium heat. Add the onion and garlic and sauté for 5–6 minutes.

2. Add the onion and garlic to a large mixing bowl. Add in the spinach, feta cheese, eggs, salt, and pepper.

3. Unroll the filo dough. Using one sheet at a time while keeping the remaining filo dough stack under a clean towel, carefully lift 1 filo dough sheet into the prepared pan and spray with the cooking spray, taking care to coat the edges of the filo, but don't overspray. Repeat this 12 times with 12 sheets of filo stacked on top of each other fitted into the pan. Spread the spinach mixture on top of the 12 sheets. Repeat with another 12 sheets stacked on top of each other, spraying each time with butter-flavored cooking spray.

4. Using a sharp knife, cut through the filo into 2 × 2 inch squares going about 1/3 down into the filo (do not cut all the way through to the bottom of the pan). Cover the pan with foil and bake for 25 minutes.

5. Remove the cover and continue to bake the spinach pie until the top is well browned and the filo dough looks crisp and flaky.

Exchanges/Choices

1 Starch
1/2 Fat

Calories	100	**Cholesterol**	20 mg	**Total Carbohydrate**	16 g
Calories from Fat	25	**Sodium**	200 mg	Dietary Fiber	2 g
Total Fat	3.0 g	**Potassium**	170 mg	Sugars	1 g
Saturated Fat	1.0 g			**Protein**	4 g
Trans Fat	0.0 g			**Phosphorus**	65 mg

RAVIOLI, ASPARAGUS, AND CHERRY TOMATO SALAD

Servings: 5	Serving Size: 3/4 cup	Prep Time: 15 minutes	Cook Time: 10 minutes

Looking for a change of pace from the usual picnic macaroni salad? This is it. Lower-fat stuffed pasta is tossed with a rainbow of colors from asparagus, cherry tomatoes, and yellow peppers. Pack this salad and toss macaroni salad to the side.

1 (9-ounce) package	frozen light cheese ravioli or other light pasta such as tortellini
1 (8-ounce) package	frozen asparagus tips
1 cup	halved salad bar cherry tomatoes
8	rehydrated sun-dried tomatoes, sliced (not oil packed)
2 whole	canned roasted yellow peppers, drained, patted dry, thinly sliced
8	halved pitted black olives

Vinaigrette

2 tablespoons	red wine vinegar
1 teaspoon	Dijon mustard
1	garlic clove, minced
	pinch sugar
1 1/2 tablespoons	olive oil

1. Bring a large pot of lightly salted water to a boil. Add in the ravioli and cook according to package directions. In the last 2 minutes, add the asparagus tips and continue to cook until both pasta and asparagus are tender. Drain gently.

2. Mix the ravioli and asparagus together with the cherry tomatoes, sun-dried tomatoes, roasted yellow peppers, and olives. Mix gently.

3. In a small bowl, whisk together the vinegar, mustard, garlic, and sugar. Slowly whisk in the olive oil until the dressing is emulsified. Add the dressing to the ravioli mixture and toss gently. Serve the salad at room temperature.

Exchanges/Choices

1 Starch	**Calories**	170	**Cholesterol**	20 mg	**Total Carbohydrate**	21 g
1 Vegetable	Calories from Fat	70	**Sodium**	280 mg	Dietary Fiber	3 g
1 1/2 Fat	**Total Fat**	8.0 g	**Potassium**	400 mg	Sugars	5 g
	Saturated Fat	2.5 g			**Protein**	7 g
	Trans Fat	0.0 g			**Phosphorus**	115 mg

SPICED SHRIMP WITH YOGURT SAUCE

A blanket of creamy yogurt covers these tender Indian spiced shrimp. Try substituting frozen and thawed chicken breasts for the shrimp.

8 ounces	plain, non-fat Greek yogurt, stirred
2 tablespoons	minced cilantro
1/2 teaspoon	ground cumin
1/4 teaspoon	ground coriander
1 tablespoon	olive oil
2	garlic cloves, minced
10 ounces	frozen peeled and deveined frozen shrimp, thawed and patted dry
1 1/2 teaspoon	garam masala
1/4 teaspoon	freshly ground black pepper

1. In a small bowl, mix together the yogurt, cilantro, cumin, and coriander, and set aside.

2. Heat the olive oil in a large skillet over medium-high heat. Add the garlic and sauté for 30 seconds. Add the shrimp, sprinkle with the garam masala and pepper, and cook for about 5–6 minutes or until the shrimp turn pink and are no longer translucent. Serve the shrimp with the yogurt sauce.

Exchanges/Choices

2 Lean Meat						
1/2 Fat	**Calories**	120	**Cholesterol**	95 mg	**Total Carbohydrate**	4 g
	Calories from Fat	40	**Sodium**	450 mg	Dietary Fiber	0 g
	Total Fat	4.5 g	**Potassium**	165 mg	Sugars	2 g
	Saturated Fat	0.7 g			**Protein**	16 g
	Trans Fat	0.0 g			**Phosphorus**	220 mg

CHICKEN PEA CURRY

Servings: 6	Serving Size: 1 cup	Prep Time: 20 minutes	Cook Time: 16 minutes

Spice up tonight's chicken with Thai-inspired ingredients. First, take a spin through the frozen section of the market and gather your chicken, onion, and peas. Add a few shelf-stable ingredients and you've created an exotic tasting main dish quickly and easily.

1 tablespoon	vegetable oil
3/4 pound	boneless, skinless chicken breasts, cut into 1-inch cubes, fresh or frozen, thawed
1 medium	onion, diced, or 1 cup frozen chopped onions
2	garlic cloves, minced
1 tablespoon	grated ginger
2 large	carrots, peeled and sliced diagonally into 1/4-inch pieces, or from the salad bar
1 medium	red pepper, cored, seeded and sliced into strips, or from salad bar
2 tablespoons	red curry paste
1/4 teaspoon	sea salt
1/4 teaspoon	freshly ground black pepper
1 (10-ounce) package	frozen peas
3/4 cup	lite coconut milk
1/2 cup	water

Garnish

sprigs of cilantro, if desired

1. Heat the oil in a large skillet or wok over medium-high heat. Add the chicken cubes and onion and sauté for 5–6 minutes until the chicken is cooked through. Remove the chicken from the pan with a slotted spoon. Add in the garlic and ginger, and sauté for 1 minute.

2. Add in the onions, carrots, and red pepper and sauté for 4 minutes until carrots and red pepper are tender. Add in the curry paste, salt, and pepper and sauté for 1 minute, coating the vegetables with the paste.

3. Add in the peas, coconut milk, and water and simmer for 3 minutes. Add back the chicken and heat through for 1 minute. Garnish with cilantro, if desired.

Exchanges/Choices

1/2 Starch	**Calories**	185	**Cholesterol**	35 mg	**Total Carbohydrate**	17 g
2 Vegetable	Calories from Fat	55	**Sodium**	370 mg	Dietary Fiber	5 g
2 Lean Meat	**Total Fat**	6.0 g	**Potassium**	450 mg	Sugars	7 g
1/2 Fat	Saturated Fat	2.4 g			**Protein**	16 g
	Trans Fat	0.0 g			**Phosphorus**	190 mg

SEARED CHICKEN WITH WINTER SQUASH SAUCE

Servings: 4   Serving Size: 1 breast, 1/3 cup sauce   Prep Time: 8-10 minutes   Cook Time: 25 minutes

Winter squash is more than a side vegetable; it makes a great sauce! Mixed with creamy ricotta cheese and aromatic shallots and garlic, you can dress up plain chicken anytime with a visit to your grocer's frozen veggie section.

1 pound	boneless, skinless chicken breasts
1/2 teaspoon	kosher salt
1/4 teaspoon	sweet paprika
1/4 teaspoon	freshly ground black pepper
1 1/2 tablespoons	olive oil, divided
2 large	shallots, minced
2	garlic cloves, minced
1/2 teaspoon	dried thyme leaves
1 (10-ounce) package	frozen winter squash puree, thawed
1/2 cup	non-fat ricotta cheese
1/4 cup	freshly grated Parmesan cheese
1/3 cup	low-fat, reduced-sodium chicken broth or water
pinch	fresh grated nutmeg
1 tablespoon	fresh lemon juice

1. Sprinkle the chicken with salt, paprika, and ground black pepper. Heat 1 tablespoon of the olive oil in a large skillet over medium-high heat.

2. Sear the chicken for 6–7 minutes per side or until cooked through. Remove the chicken to a plate, tent with foil to keep warm.

3. Add the remaining 1/2 tablespoon of oil to the pan. Add in the shallot, garlic, and thyme and sauté for 2 minutes. Add in the squash puree, ricotta cheese, Parmesan cheese, broth or water, and nutmeg. Simmer on low heat for about 4–5 minutes until heated through. Add in the lemon juice. Taste and correct the seasonings. Serve the chicken with the winter squash sauce.

Exchanges/Choices

1/2 Starch	**Calories**	260	**Cholesterol**	80 mg	**Total Carbohydrate**	12 g
1 Vegetable	Calories from Fat	80	**Sodium**	440 mg	Dietary Fiber	2 g
4 Lean Meat	**Total Fat**	9.0 g	**Potassium**	420 mg	Sugars	3 g
1/2 Fat	Saturated Fat	2.2 g			**Protein**	31 g
	Trans Fat	0.0 g			**Phosphorus**	290 mg

SALMON WITH BLUEBERRY SALSA

Servings: 4   Serving Size: 4 oz. salmon, 1/4 cup salsa   Prep Time: 10 minutes   Cook Time: 17 minutes

There's tomato salsa and then there's blueberry salsa! For your next meal, there's no need to wait till summer for fresh blueberries when frozen are at hand. Mixed with red onion and red pepper with a hint of heat from jalapeño peppers, this salsa's gorgeous color contrasts very nicely with the pretty pink salmon.

Salsa

1 cup	frozen blueberries, thawed and drained
1/4 cup	minced red onion
1/4 cup	minced red bell pepper
1/2 small	jalapeño pepper, seeded and minced
2 tablespoons	fresh lime juice
2 teaspoons	honey
1 pound	salmon filets, fresh or frozen, thawed
1 tablespoon	olive oil
1/2 teaspoon	Kosher salt
1/4 teaspoon	freshly ground black pepper

1. Combine all the blueberry salsa ingredients in a bowl. Mix gently. Cover and set aside at room temperature.

2. Preheat the oven to 400 degrees. Line a broiler pan with foil. Coat the foil with cooking spray. Add the salmon filets to the pan and brush each filet with the oil. Sprinkle with salt and pepper.

3. Roast the salmon for about 10–12 minutes. Position the broiler tray about 4–5 inches from the heat source and turn the oven to broil. Broil the salmon for about 2–3 minutes until golden. Drain any excess liquid from the salsa and serve with salmon.

Exchanges/Choices

1/2 Carbohydrate	**Calories**	270	**Cholesterol**	80 mg	**Total Carbohydrate**	11 g
4 Lean Meat	Calories from Fat	125	**Sodium**	305 mg	Dietary Fiber	2 g
1 Fat	**Total Fat**	14.0 g	**Potassium**	430 mg	Sugars	7 g
	Saturated Fat	2.3 g			**Protein**	26 g
	Trans Fat	0.0 g			**Phosphorus**	270 mg

EASY ITALIAN SKILLET

Servings: 8   **Serving Size:** 2 oz. pasta, 1/2 cup sauce   **Prep Time:** 15 minutes   **Cook Time:** 40 minutes

Got some extra ground beef in the freezer? Get creative and turn it into this one-pot easy skillet. Visit the freezer section of the market to pick up the multicolored pepper medley and then add some shelf-staple products, and voila: dinner is done!

3/4 pound	lean (at least 90%) ground beef, fresh or frozen, thawed
2 teaspoons	olive oil
2 cups	sliced mushrooms (from the salad bar or produce section)
1 (10-ounce) package	frozen onion and bell pepper medley, thawed, drained, and patted lightly dry
3	garlic cloves, minced
1 1/2 teaspoons	dried basil
1 1/2 teaspoons	dried oregano
1/3 cup	dry red wine
1 (14.5-ounce) can	diced fire-roasted tomatoes, undrained
1/4 teaspoon	Kosher salt
1/4 teaspoon	freshly ground black pepper
	pinch sugar
	pinch crushed dried red chili flakes
8 ounces	whole-wheat penne pasta
1/4 cup	fresh grated Parmesan cheese (optional)

1. Heat a large skillet over medium-high heat. Add the ground beef and cook, breaking up the meat, for about 5–6 minutes until the meat is no longer pink. Remove the meat with a slotted spoon to a bowl and set aside.

2. Drain any excess fat from the skillet. Add the olive oil and mushrooms to the skillet and sauté the mushrooms for about 4–5 minutes just until they brown and are about to give up their liquid. Remove the mushrooms from the skillet to a bowl and set aside. Add in the onion and bell pepper medley and garlic and sauté for 4 minutes. Add in the basil and oregano and sauté for 1 minute.

3. Add back the mushrooms and add in the red wine. Cook over medium heat until the wine is almost evaporated. Add in the tomatoes, salt, black pepper, sugar, red chili flakes and reserved ground beef. Lower the heat to simmer and cook for about 15–20 minutes.

4. Meanwhile, bring a large pot of lightly salted water to boil. Add in the penne pasta and cook for about 7–9 minutes or until al dente. Drain. Add the pasta to the sauce and toss well. Serve with Parmesan cheese if desired.

Exchanges/Choices

1 1/2 Starch	**Calories**	215	**Cholesterol**	25 mg	**Total Carbohydrate**	28 g
1 Vegetable	Calories from Fat	45	**Sodium**	225 mg	Dietary Fiber	4 g
1 Lean Meat	**Total Fat**	5.0 g	**Potassium**	365 mg	Sugars	3 g
1/2 Fat	Saturated Fat	1.6 g			**Protein**	13 g
	Trans Fat	0.2 g			**Phosphorus**	160 mg

BROWN RICE AND EDAMAME SALAD

Servings: 5   **Serving Size:** 1 cup   **Prep Time:** 10 minutes   **Cook Time:** 12 minutes

My new favorite frozen product is edamame. It is only widely available in frozen form. Stock up with edamame, pair it with frozen brown rice, and you can have a really healthy meal in about 10 minutes.

1 1/2 cups	frozen edamame, thawed
1/4 cup	raisins or currants
2 tablespoons	fresh lime juice
1/2 teaspoon	sugar
2 teaspoons	vegetable oil
1	onion, diced
1	garlic clove, minced
1 tablespoon	fresh grated ginger
1/2 teaspoon	curry powder
1/2 teaspoon	Kosher salt
1/4 teaspoon	freshly ground black pepper
2 cups	frozen long-grain brown rice, cooked and cooled
2 tablespoons	fresh minced cilantro

1 Add the thawed edamame to a strainer and let drain thoroughly of all moisture. Pat dry and set aside.

2 In a small bowl, combine the raisins, lime juice, and sugar and set aside.

3 Heat the vegetable oil in a medium skillet over medium-high heat. Add the onion and sauté for about 6 minutes. Add the garlic and sauté for 2 minutes. Add in the ginger, curry, salt, and pepper and sauté for 2 minutes. Remove the skillet from the heat and add in the raisin mixture and mix.

4 Add the cooked rice and reserved edamame to a serving bowl. Add in the onion mixture and cilantro. Mix gently. Serve the salad at room temperature.

Exchanges/Choices

1 1/2 Starch	**Calories**	185	**Cholesterol**	0 mg	**Total Carbohydrate**	30 g
1/2 Fruit	Calories from Fat	45	**Sodium**	200 mg	Dietary Fiber	5 g
1 Lean Meat	**Total Fat**	5.0 g	**Potassium**	345 mg	Sugars	7 g
	Saturated Fat	0.6 g			**Protein**	7 g
	Trans Fat	0.0 g			**Phosphorus**	150 mg

PENNE WITH SPICED SHRIMP AND BROCCOLI

Servings: 8   Serving Size: 1 cup   Prep Time: 5 minutes   Cook Time: 15 minutes

We often think of pasta as having to be smothered it in tomato sauce. Not so. One of the most important lessons I learned in Italy was that pasta could be mixed with a myriad of fresh vegetables, garlic, herbs, and spices without ever including tomato sauce.

8 ounces	whole-wheat penne pasta
2 teaspoons	sweet paprika
1 teaspoon	dried basil
1 teaspoon	garlic powder
1/2 teaspoon	dried thyme leaves
1/4 teaspoon	Kosher salt
1/4 teaspoon	fresh ground black pepper
1/8 teaspoon	cayenne pepper
3/4 pound	large frozen shrimp, peeled and deveined, thawed and patted dry
1 1/2 tablespoons	olive oil, divided
1/2 cup	chopped onion
3	garlic cloves, minced
1 (10-ounce) package	frozen broccoli florets, slightly thawed
1/4 cup	grated fresh Parmesan cheese
1/4 cup	chopped jarred roasted red peppers, drained well and patted dry
	juice of 1/2 lemon

1. Bring a large pot of lightly salted water to a boil. Add the penne and cook for about 7–9 minutes just until al dente.

2. Meanwhile, mix together the paprika, basil, garlic powder, thyme, salt, pepper, and cayenne pepper in a large bowl. Add in the shrimp and toss to coat well.

3. Heat 1 tablespoon of the oil in a large skillet, add the shrimp, and cook for about 4–5 minutes, just until the shrimp are cooked through. Remove the shrimp from the skillet. Add the remaining 1/2 tablespoon of oil and sauté the onion and garlic for 4 minutes. Add the broccoli florets and sauté for another 4 minutes until broccoli is cooked through. Add the shrimp back to the skillet.

4. Drain the pasta and toss the shrimp mixture with the pasta. Sprinkle with Parmesan cheese and roasted red peppers. Drizzle with the lemon juice.

Exchanges/Choices

1 1/2 Starch	**Calories**	205	**Cholesterol**	70 mg	**Total Carbohydrate**	27 g
1 Vegetable	Calories from Fat	40	**Sodium**	480 mg	Dietary Fiber	4 g
1 Lean Meat	**Total Fat**	4.5 g	**Potassium**	255 mg	Sugars	3 g
1/2 Fat	Saturated Fat	0.9 g			**Protein**	14 g
	Trans Fat	0.0 g			**Phosphorus**	190 mg

VEGETARIAN SKILLET

Servings: 4   Serving Size: 1 cup   Prep Time: 10 minutes   Cook Time: 18 minutes

Finding fresh lima beans is a challenge, so I love that frozen ones are available anytime. This one-pot skillet dish is reminiscent of succotash but with the addition of extra fiber from chickpeas. One pot, less than 20 minutes to prepare, what could be better?

1 tablespoon	olive oil
1/2 cup	diced onion
2	garlic cloves, minced
1/2 small	jalapeño pepper, seeded and minced
1 cup	frozen lima beans
1 cup	frozen corn
1 (14.5-ounce) can	fire roasted tomatoes, drained
1 cup	canned chickpeas, drained and rinsed
1/2 teaspoon	Kosher salt
1/4 teaspoon	freshly ground black pepper

Garnish

1/4 cup	fat-free sour cream

1. Heat the oil in a large skillet over medium heat. Add the onion and sauté for 4 minutes. Add the garlic and jalapeño and sauté for 2 minutes.

2. Add in the lima beans and corn and cook until the beans are tender, about 10 minutes. Add in the tomatoes, chickpeas, salt, and pepper and cook for 2 minutes.

3. Serve with a dollop of sour cream.

Exchanges/Choices

2 Starch	**Calories**	205	**Cholesterol**	0 mg	**Total Carbohydrate**	34 g
1 Lean Meat	Calories from Fat	45	**Sodium**	505 mg	Dietary Fiber	7 g
	Total Fat	5.0 g	**Potassium**	525 mg	Sugars	7 g
	Saturated Fat	0.7 g			**Protein**	8 g
	Trans Fat	0.0 g			**Phosphorus**	170 mg

WINTER SQUASH POLENTA

| Servings: 4 | Serving Size: 2/3 cup | Prep Time: 5 minutes | Cook Time: 20 minutes |

There are so many great dishes to warm the bones on a chilly evening, but one of my all-time favorites is a bowl of creamy polenta. Here, I've added oh-so-convenient frozen pureed winter squash to make this cornmeal-based comfort dish rich and filling. A touch of golden maple syrup provides just the right balance to further bring out winter squash's special natural sweetness.

4 cups	water
1 cup	coarse polenta
1/2 teaspoon	sea salt
1/4 teaspoon	freshly ground black pepper
1 cup	thawed frozen winter squash puree
1 tablespoon	pure maple syrup

Garnish

1/4 cup	grated fresh Parmesan cheese

1. In a medium saucepan, bring the water to a boil. Add the polenta, salt, and pepper and whisk on medium-low heat until the polenta is thickened and comes away from the sides of the pan, about 15 minutes.

2. Add in the winter squash and maple syrup. Season with salt and pepper. Garnish with the Parmesan cheese.

Exchanges/Choices

2 1/2 Starch

Calories	185	**Cholesterol**	5 mg	**Total Carbohydrate**	36 g
Calories from Fat	15	**Sodium**	380 mg	Dietary Fiber	3 g
Total Fat	1.5 g	**Potassium**	145 mg	Sugars	4 g
Saturated Fat	0.8 g			**Protein**	5 g
Trans Fat	0.0 g			**Phosphorus**	75 mg

CURRIED RICE WITH SHRIMP AND BASIL

Servings: 4   Serving Size: 1 cup   Prep Time: 10 minutes   Cook Time: 20 minutes

Brown rice is now available already cooked and frozen. All you need to do is add it to your favorite dish. Gone are the days where you had to wait an hour for fluffy, cooked brown rice. Just reheat and serve! This pungent curried shrimp dish can be on your table in less than 30 minutes.

1 tablespoon	olive oil
1 large	onion, chopped
2	garlic cloves, minced
2 teaspoons	curry powder
2 cups	frozen, cooked brown rice
1/3 cup	low-fat, reduced-sodium chicken broth
12 ounces	frozen, cooked, peeled and deveined shrimp, thawed and patted dry
1/4 teaspoon	freshly ground black pepper
1/2 cup	fresh sliced basil
1/4 to 1/2 teaspoon	hot sauce

1. Heat the oil in a large skillet over medium heat. Add in the onion and garlic and sauté for 6–7 minutes. Add in the curry powder and sauté for 1 minute.

2. Add in the frozen brown rice, breaking up any large chunks (if the rice is frozen solid, microwave the rice until it can be broken up into pieces). Sauté the rice for 3 minutes. Add in the broth and cover and cook until broth is absorbed and the rice is tender. Add in the shrimp and pepper and cook until the shrimp is heated through, about 2–3 minutes.

3. Add in the basil and hot sauce. Serve.

Exchanges/Choices

1 1/2 Starch	**Calories**	215	**Cholesterol**	115 mg	**Total Carbohydrate**	27 g
1 Vegetable	Calories from Fat	45	**Sodium**	565 mg	Dietary Fiber	3 g
1 Lean Meat	**Total Fat**	5.0 g	**Potassium**	275 mg	Sugars	3 g
1/2 Fat	Saturated Fat	0.9 g			**Protein**	16 g
	Trans Fat	0.0 g			**Phosphorus**	265 mg

CHAPTER 6

Cans, Boxes, and Jars
From the Shelves

Imagine simply picking a few items off the shelf in your pantry and assembling them into a simple flavorful and healthy meal for you and your family. If your pantry is well stocked, there is no need for daily grocery store stops. There are countless canned, boxed, and jarred foods that are tremendously convenient and healthful and should be incorporated into your everyday cooking.

The word pantry derives from the French word, panetiere or the "bread room." This term was used as far back as 1250 A.D. I imagine that the bread room was filled with sacks of flour, preserved fruits and vegetables, possibly condiments, and dried herbs and spices. It was commonplace to have a well stocked pantry because you never knew when there would be a food shortage and grocery stores were not on every corner.

We can learn a great deal about how to stock our pantry from 13th century practices. Fast forward to today's modern pantry and you will discover that your pantry can go way further than our ancestors' pantry. If you stock your pantry as I suggest, you will be able to mix and match standbys for hundreds of easy meals. As your interest in cooking expands, so will your pantry. For example once you have the basic vinegars on hand, branch out to include the more exotic kinds, such as Champagne vinegar. Extra virgin olive oil is easy to find, but perhaps you'll want to add walnut or macadamia nut oil to the shelf to create wonderfully aromatic dishes.

A PANTRY IS A WORK IN PROGRESS. You don't need to fill it up in one fell swoop. Here is a guide to the items you should have on hand in your pantry, listing most of the ingredients used in this section's recipes.

Must Have Basics for a Well-Stocked Pantry

The following basic items can be stored up to 1 year in the pantry. Store brown rice and whole-grain pastas in airtight containers. Avoid purchasing any dented cans or bottles.

Canned Beans: black, pinto, chickpea, and red kidney. Leftover canned beans can be stored in the refrigerator in an airtight container for 2–3 days. Whenever possible look for canned beans and other canned products that are BPA free. Use up canned foods quickly and never store leftovers in the can itself. If you prefer to soak and cook your own beans, you will find a good assortment of dried beans on your grocers shelf.

Canned Tuna and Salmon: any leftover canned fish can be stored in the refrigerator in an airtight container for 1–2 days.

Brown Rice: Store brown rice with a dried red chile pepper to keep it fresh. It also keeps any mealy bugs away. Cooked brown rice can be stored in an airtight container for up to 1 week. Also, look for convenient already cooked brown rice that comes in 1 cup portions; a real time saver!

Whole Grain Pasta: When uncooked boxed pasta develops white speckles, toss. Cooked pasta can be stored in an airtight container for up to 2–3 days for best freshness.

Fat-Free, Reduced-Sodium Chicken and Vegetable Broths: Broth is for more than just a soup base. Use broth for making sauces, cooking grains and pasta, and for a flavor boost instead of plain water. Sauté vegetables in broth for fat-free cooking. Once boxed broth is opened, reseal, store in the refrigerator, and use within 1–2 weeks.

Whole and Diced Tomatoes: Fresh tomatoes have a short season. Open a can of whole tomatoes and crush them coarsely in your hands. Use a base for homemade pasta sauce. Add canned diced tomatoes to top a grilled chicken breast or add to soups for a heartier texture. Store any leftover canned tomatoes in an airtight container and refrigerate for 3–4 days. You can freeze canned tomatoes in an airtight container for up to 4–5 months for best freshness.

Tomato Paste: Although slightly more expensive, purchase tomato paste in the convenient tubes rather than the can. Leftover tomato paste is more easily stored in a tube than in the can.

Flavor Boosters

Vinegar: Red, White, Balsamic: Use within 1 year. Can be stored in pantry or refrigerator.

Extra Virgin Olive Oil: Transfer oil to a dark opaque container. Use within 6–7 months for best freshness.

Low Sodium Soy Sauce: Use within 1 year. Can also be stored in the refrigerator.

Dijon Mustard: Use within 1 year. Once opened, store in the refrigerator.

Salsa: Add salsa to rice as it cooks, top a grilled fish filet, or use as a sauce for cooked vegetables. Keep for 1 year in pantry. Once opened, keep in refrigerator for no more than 1 month.

Fresh Onions and Garlic: Store these in the bottom of the pantry in a container that provides air circulation. Onions and garlic will store for 1–2 weeks. If they start to sprout, time to toss.

Dried Herbs and Spices: Keep away from light and heat. Use dried herbs and spices within 1 year for best freshness. Make sure lids are tightly sealed.

Capers: Use within 1 year. Once opened, store in refrigerator and use within 2 months.

Olives: Use within 1 year. Once opened, store in the refrigerator and use within a few weeks.

No-Sugar-Added Preserves: Use these preserves for more than just toast. Use as part of a glaze for pan-seared meat, chicken, or fish. Melt it down for syrup for pancakes, waffles, and French toast. Use within 1 year. Once opened, store in the refrigerator and use within 8–9 months.

Plain Breadcrumbs: Preferably the coarse-cut Japanese panko breadcrumbs, which are easily found in most markets. Store in a tightly covered container and use within 1 year.

A Few Exotics

Although not really as exotic as they were years ago, I've included some delicious canned and bottled condiments that will really add sparkle to your foods. Think about having these on hand as well.

Hoisin Sauce

Red or Brown Miso

Lite Coconut Milk

Pesto Sauce

Dried Wild Mushrooms

Sun-Dried Tomatoes

Red Curry Paste

GINGER PORK

Servings: 4
Marinating Time: 8 hours
Serving Size: 1 pork chop
Cook Time: 15 minutes
Prep Time: 5 minutes

Whenever I dine out at Asian restaurants, my eye is first drawn to any dish that has ginger. This all-purpose marinade is overflowing with warm, spicy ginger and has so many flavor notes, you will not believe something so good comes from just simple staple ingredients.

4 (5–6 ounce)	bone-in lean pork chops (about 1/2-inch thick)
3 tablespoons	light soy sauce
3 tablespoons	rice vinegar
1 tablespoon	honey
1 tablespoon	peeled, grated fresh minced ginger
3	garlic cloves, minced
2 teaspoons	toasted sesame oil
1/4 teaspoon	crushed red pepper flakes

1 Trim any excess fat from the pork chops.

2 In a zippered plastic bag, combine the soy sauce, vinegar, honey, ginger, garlic, sesame oil, and red pepper flakes. Add in the pork chops. Seal the bag and mix the marinade over the pork chops.

3 Refrigerate the pork for at least 8 hours or overnight.

4 Preheat an oven broiler with the rack set 4 inches from the heat source. Cover a broiler pan with foil. Coat the foil with cooking spray. Or set an outdoor grill to high heat. Coat the rack with cooking spray.

5 Remove the pork chops from the marinade, pour the excess marinade into a small saucepan, and set aside. Add the pork chops to the prepared broiler pan or add directly onto the grill rack.

6 Broil or grill the pork for about 5–6 minutes per side or until cooked through. Meanwhile, heat the reserved marinade over medium high heat. Bring to a boil, reduce the heat, and simmer for 5 minutes.

7 Serve the pork chops with the reserved heated marinade.

Exchanges/Choices

1/2 Carbohydrate	**Calories**	195	**Cholesterol**	60 mg	**Total Carbohydrate**	7 g	
3 Lean Meat	Calories from Fat	70	**Sodium**	455 mg	Dietary Fiber	0 g	
1/2 Fat	**Total Fat**	8.0 g	**Potassium**	300 mg	Sugars	5 g	
	Saturated Fat	2.5 g			**Protein**	22 g	
	Trans Fat	0.0 g			**Phosphorus**	145 mg	

SALSA FLANK STEAK

One of the "tricks" I learned from a mentor years ago was to take commercially prepared healthy foods and give them a flavor boost with a few additional ingredients. Here I take your favorite salsa and zip it up with garlic, onion, and basil. You do half the work and get twice the taste!

1 tablespoon	garlic flavored olive oil
1 small	onion, minced
1	garlic clove, finely minced
1 cup	bottled mild or hot salsa
1 tablespoon	red wine vinegar
1 tablespoon	fresh minced basil (optional)
1 pound	lean flank steak
1/2 teaspoon	Kosher salt
	freshly ground black pepper to taste

1. Heat the oil in a large skillet over medium heat. Add in the onion and garlic and sauté for 3–4 minutes until onion just turns translucent.

2. Add in the salsa and vinegar and cook for 5 minutes. Add in the basil if using. Turn off the heat and set aside.

3. Meanwhile, sprinkle the flank steak on one side with salt and pepper. With a sharp knife, make three diagonal slashes in the flank steak set a few inches apart. This will prevent the flank steak from curling up as it cooks.

4. Preheat an oven broiler with the rack set 4 inches from the heat source. Cover a broiler pan with foil. Coat the foil with cooking spray. Or set an outdoor grill to high heat. Coat the rack with cooking spray.

5. Add the steak to the prepared pan or set directly on the grill. Broil or grill the steak for about 6–8 minutes per side or until desired degree of doneness. Remove the steak from the broiler or grill and set aside on a carving board for 5 minutes to let juices settle.

6. Slice the flank steak diagonally across the grain into thin slices. Serve the steak with the salsa.

Exchanges/Choices

1 Vegetable	**Calories**	140	**Cholesterol**	25 mg	**Total Carbohydrate**	4 g
2 Lean Meat	Calories from Fat	55	**Sodium**	440 mg	Dietary Fiber	1 g
1/2 Fat	**Total Fat**	6.0 g	**Potassium**	340 mg	Sugars	2 g
	Saturated Fat	2.0 g			**Protein**	16 g
	Trans Fat	0.0 g			**Phosphorus**	135 mg

ORANGE RAISIN PORK LOIN CHOPS

I'm always looking for dishes that do double duty; a good everyday dish that can also be served when I entertain. A great entertaining dish has to have a heavenly aroma, and an elegant look, yet be easy enough to prepare so I can actually enjoy being with my guests. Not only can you serve this pork chop recipe on weekdays, but your guests will be impressed with this jewel like sauce smothered all over sweet and spicy coated lean pork.

1 tablespoon	flour
1 tablespoon	brown sugar (or brown sugar substitute)
1/2 teaspoon	ground cumin
1/2 teaspoon	ground coriander
1/4 teaspoon	ground red pepper
1/4 teaspoon	Kosher salt
1/4 teaspoon	freshly ground black pepper
4 (4-ounce)	boneless pork loin chops
1/4 cup	fresh orange juice
3 tablespoons	good quality balsamic vinegar
3 tablespoons	raisins
1 tablespoon	vegetable oil

1 Combine the flour, brown sugar, cumin, coriander, red pepper, salt, and pepper on a large plate. Dredge each pork loin chop in the spice mixture, shaking off any excess. Add the pork chops to a clean plate and set aside.

2 In a small bowl, combine the orange juice, vinegar, and raisins. Set aside.

3 Heat the oil in a large skillet over medium-high heat. Add the pork loin chops and sear on both sides for about 3 minutes per side. Add in the orange juice-raisin mixture and cook until the sauce thickens and the pork chops are cooked through.

Exchanges/Choices

1 Carbohydrate	**Calories**	245	**Cholesterol**	60 mg	**Total Carbohydrate**	14 g
3 Lean Meat	Calories from Fat	100	**Sodium**	170 mg	Dietary Fiber	0 g
1 Fat	**Total Fat**	11.0 g	**Potassium**	410 mg	Sugars	10 g
	Saturated Fat	2.8 g			**Protein**	22 g
	Trans Fat	0.0 g			**Phosphorus**	190 mg

ROASTED PEPPER PENNE

| Servings: 8 | Serving Size: 1 cup | Prep Time: 5 minutes | Cook Time: 20 minutes |

When I have the time, I will indeed roast sweet bell peppers. But I love them so much that I want them ready when I am. To the rescue come convenient roasted bell peppers in the jar that make this penne dish simply gorgeous. Dotted with juicy olives and a touch of prosciutto, all the flavors and textures work together so well, I can see this as your go-to dish often!

4 large	jarred roasted red peppers, drained well and patted dry
4 large	roasted jarred yellow peppers, drained well and patted dry
1/4 cup	pitted, chopped Kalamata olives
2 teaspoons	capers
1 1/2 tablespoons	olive oil
2 ounces	sliced prosciutto, cut into thin strips
8 ounces	whole-wheat penne
1/4 cup	fresh minced parsley
1 teaspoon	grated lemon zest
2 tablespoons	grated fresh Parmesan cheese

1 Bring a large pot of lightly salted water to a boil. Meanwhile, slice the red and yellow roasted peppers into thin strips. Add to a bowl. Add in the olives, capers, and olive oil. Set aside.

2 Cook the prosciutto in a large skillet over medium high heat just until crisp. Remove the prosciutto from the pan and set aside. Add the pepper mixture to the pan and cook over low heat for 3–4 minutes.

3 Meanwhile, add the penne to the boiling water and cook the penne about 7–8 minutes or until al dente. Drain. Toss the pepper sauce and pasta together. Top with reserved prosciutto, parsley, lemon zest, and Parmesan cheese.

Exchanges/Choices

1 1/2 Starch	**Calories**	185	**Cholesterol**	5 mg	**Total Carbohydrate**	28 g
1 Vegetable	Calories from Fat	55	**Sodium**	340 mg	Dietary Fiber	4 g
1 Fat	**Total Fat**	6.0 g	**Potassium**	200 mg	Sugars	5 g
	Saturated Fat	1.0 g			**Protein**	7 g
	Trans Fat	0.0 g			**Phosphorus**	95 mg

ZESTY BBQ CHICKEN

Servings: 4   Serving Size: 2 thighs   Prep Time: 5 minutes   Cook Time: 45 minutes

When your pantry is properly stocked with the ingredients you really use, there is no limit to making meals nutritious and easy. Get out those common spices and herbs to create this juicy barbecued chicken recipe. It's all so good to the very last messy bite.

Spice rub

1 tablespoon	brown sugar
1 tablespoon	sweet paprika
2 teaspoons	garlic powder
1 teaspoon	onion powder
1/2 teaspoon	celery seed
1/2 teaspoon	Kosher salt
1/2 teaspoon	ground black pepper
1/4 teaspoon	cayenne pepper
1 1/2 pounds	skinless chicken thighs

Sauce

1 cup	low-sodium ketchup
2 tablespoons	cider vinegar
1 tablespoon	Worcestershire sauce
1 tablespoon	brown sugar (or sugar substitute)
1 tablespoon	Dijon mustard
1 teaspoon	liquid smoke
1/4 teaspoon	ground black pepper

1 Combine all the ingredients for the spice rub. Rub all over the chicken thighs. Add the chicken to a plate and set aside.

2 Meanwhile, combine all the ingredients for the sauce in a saucepan. Bring to a boil over medium-high heat. Reduce the heat to simmer and cook for 15–20 minutes until sauce is thick and dark.

3 Heat an outdoor grill to medium-high heat. Coat the rack with cooking spray. Add the chicken and cook over direct heat for about 20 minutes, turning once. Brush on half of the sauce and continue to cook the chicken for about 10–15 minutes until the chicken is cooked through. Serve remaining heated sauce on the side.

Exchanges/Choices

1 1/2 Carbohydrate
3 Lean Meat

Calories	255	
Calories from Fat	70	
Total Fat	8.0	g
Saturated Fat	2.0	g
Trans Fat	0.0	g

Cholesterol	115	mg
Sodium	465	mg
Potassium	585	mg

Total Carbohydrate	26	g
Dietary Fiber	1	g
Sugars	22	g
Protein	22	g
Phosphorus	225	mg

MISO SALMON

Servings: 4   **Serving Size:** 4 ounces
Prep Time: 1 hour and 5 minutes (includes marinating time)   **Cook Time:** 8–10 minutes

It's always fun to add something new to your ingredient list especially if it packs a punch of flavor. One of my favorite "unusual" ingredients to keep on hand is miso. Made from fermented soy beans, miso adds a smoky depth to so many foods. It stores well in the refrigerator making it easy to access anytime. The rich flavor goes so well with salmon.

Marinade

3 tablespoons	brown rice or red miso
2 tablespoons	light soy sauce
2 tablespoons	fresh orange juice
1 tablespoon	brown sugar (or sugar substitute) or honey
1 teaspoon	grated fresh orange zest
	pinch crushed red pepper flakes
4 (4-ounce)	salmon filets

1. Combine the miso, soy sauce, orange juice, sugar, orange zest, and red pepper flakes in a large bowl. Add the salmon and turn to coat. Cover and refrigerate for 1 hour.

2. Preheat an oven broiler with the rack set 4 inches from the heat source. Cover a broiler pan with foil. Coat the foil with cooking spray. Or set an outdoor grill to high heat. Coat the rack with cooking spray.

3. Remove the salmon from the marinade, letting any excess drip back into the bowl. Discard the excess marinade. Add the salmon to the pan skin side down.

4. Broil or grill the salmon for about 8–10 minutes until desired doneness. Let the salmon rest a few minutes before serving to allow juices to settle.

Exchanges/Choices

4 Lean Meat	**Calories**	225	**Cholesterol**	80 mg	**Total Carbohydrate**	4 g
1/2 Fat	Calories from Fat	90	**Sodium**	440 mg	Dietary Fiber	1 g
	Total Fat	10.0 g	**Potassium**	375 mg	Sugars	3 g
	Saturated Fat	1.8 g			**Protein**	26 g
	Trans Fat	0.0 g			**Phosphorus**	270 mg

MUSHROOM POLENTA

Servings: 4   Serving Size: 1 cup   Prep Time: 25 minutes   Cook Time: 22 minutes

Polenta became a favorite of mine when I first visited Italy eons ago. It's so easy to prepare and when it's topped with a super easy sauce made from a bit of the salad bar and must-have shelf staple ingredients, how fast can you say ciao bella?

Sauce

1 tablespoon	olive oil
3/4 pound	salad bar mushrooms (about 3 cups)
3	garlic cloves, minced
1 teaspoon	Italian seasoning
2 cups	jarred marinara sauce
1 tablespoon	good quality balsamic vinegar

Polenta

3 cups	water
1/2 tablespoon	butter
1/4 teaspoon	Kosher salt
1/4 teaspoon	sugar
1 cup	medium coarse polenta

1. Heat the olive oil in a large skillet over high heat. Add the mushrooms and let them sit undisturbed for 2 minutes. Begin to stir the mushrooms and cook until the mushrooms are golden brown. Add in the garlic and sauté for 1 minute. When most of the water is released from the mushrooms, add in the Italian seasoning and cook 1 minute. Add in the jarred sauce and lower the heat and simmer for 10 minutes. Add in the balsamic vinegar and simmer for 2 minutes.

2. Meanwhile, prepare the polenta. Bring the water, butter, salt, and sugar to a boil in a large saucepan. In a thin steady stream, whisk in the polenta. Lower the heat to simmer and continue stirring until the polenta thickens and leaves the sides of the pan.

3. Pour the polenta into individual bowls and top with the mushroom sauce.

Exchanges/Choices

2 Starch	**Calories**	280	**Cholesterol**	5 mg	**Total Carbohydrate**	41 g
1 Vegetable	Calories from Fat	90	**Sodium**	465 mg	Dietary Fiber	5 g
2 Fat	**Total Fat**	10.0 g	**Potassium**	705 mg	Sugars	8 g
	Saturated Fat	2.0 g			**Protein**	8 g
	Trans Fat	0.1 g			**Phosphorus**	150 mg

BLACK AND WHITE BEAN SALAD

Servings: 3   Serving Size: 1 cup   Preparation Time: 10 minutes   Cook Time: 0

Just five ingredients and you have a summery salad to bring to your next picnic. The contrast of black and white beans bathed in salsa spiked with balsamic vinegar and cilantro will have everyone thinking there's more than the minimal ingredients used.

1 (15-ounce) can	black beans, drained and rinsed
1 (15-ounce) can	cannellini or white navy beans, drained and rinsed
3/4 cup	jarred mild or hot salsa
2 tablespoons	good quality balsamic vinegar
2 tablespoons	minced fresh cilantro

1 Combine all ingredients in a large bowl. Cover and refrigerate for 1 hour prior to serving. Remove from the refrigerator and bring to room temperature to serve.

Exchanges/Choices

2 1/2 Starch
1 Lean Meat

Calories	235	**Cholesterol**	0 mg	**Total Carbohydrate**	43 g
Calories from Fat	10	**Sodium**	555 mg	Dietary Fiber	13 g
Total Fat	1.0 g	**Potassium**	815 mg	Sugars	5 g
Saturated Fat	0.2 g			**Protein**	15 g
Trans Fat	0.0 g			**Phosphorus**	245 mg

CHICKEN WITH PINEAPPLE MANDARIN ORANGE SALSA

Servings: 4	Serving Size: 1 breast, 1/2 cup salsa	Prep Time: 20 minutes
Cook Time: 16 minutes	Chilling Time for Salsa: 1 hour	

When I was a kid, I actually wasn't a big fan of fresh fruit. But canned mandarin oranges always excited me and I have warm memories of a little cut glass bowl my Mom used to serve the tiny orange segments. I've of course expanded my fruit repertoire, but still think mandarin oranges are a great versatile fruit. Here, a simple salsa spiked with tropical coconut pairs well with cumin flavored seared chicken breasts.

Salsa

1 cup	pineapple tidbits packed in their own juice, well drained
1 cup	mandarin oranges packed in water or their juice, well drained, coarsely chopped
2	scallions, white part only, minced
1/4 cup	minced red bell pepper
1 1/2 tablespoons	unsweetened coconut flakes
1/4 teaspoon	crushed red pepper flakes

Chicken

1 pound	boneless, skinless chicken breasts
1 teaspoon	ground cumin
1 teaspoon	mild or hot chili powder
1/4 teaspoon	Kosher salt
	freshly ground black pepper to taste
1 tablespoon	vegetable oil

1. Line a baking sheet with foil. Preheat the oven to 375 degrees. Combine all the ingredients for the salsa in a bowl. Cover and refrigerate for 1 hour.

2. Meanwhile, trim any excess fat from the chicken breasts. Combine the cumin, chili powder, salt, and pepper. Rub each piece of chicken with the spice rub.

3. Heat the oil in a large skillet over medium-high heat. Add the chicken and sear on both sides for a total of 10 minutes. Add the chicken to the prepared baking sheet. Cover loosely with foil or parchment paper. Continue to cook the chicken breasts until cooked through, about 6–7 minutes.

4. Bring the salsa up to room temperature. Serve the cooked chicken with the salsa.

Exchanges/Choices

1 Fruit	**Calories**	225	**Cholesterol**	65 mg	**Total Carbohydrate**	14 g	
3 Lean Meat	Calories from Fat	70	**Sodium**	190 mg	Dietary Fiber	2 g	
1/2 Fat	**Total Fat**	8.0 g	**Potassium**	390 mg	Sugars	11 g	
	Saturated Fat	2.3 g			**Protein**	25 g	
	Trans Fat	0.0 g			**Phosphorus**	200 mg	

ROASTED RED PEPPER CHICKEN

Servings: 4	Serving Size: 1 breast	Prep Time: 5 minutes	Cook Time: 25 minutes

Need to impress some guests without a lot of effort. Look no further than preparing this recipe, which has all the shelf-stable products you should always keep on hand. The beautiful red colored sauce spiked with olives and capers elevates this dish to a special meal.

4 (4-ounce)	chicken breasts
1/2 teaspoon	Kosher salt
1/2 teaspoon	sweet paprika
1/4 teaspoon	freshly ground black pepper
1 tablespoon	olive oil, divided
1 teaspoon	butter
1/2 cup	dry white wine
1 medium	onion, diced
1	garlic clove, minced
3 whole	jarred roasted red peppers, drained and patted dry
1 1/2 tablespoons	evaporated fat-free milk
1 1/2 teaspoons	dried Italian seasoning
2 tablespoons	coarsely chopped pitted black olives
1 tablespoon	small capers, drained
1 teaspoon	sugar
1 tablespoon	fat-free sour cream

1. Sprinkle both sides of each chicken breast with salt, paprika, and freshly ground black pepper.

2. Heat half the olive oil and the butter in a large skillet over medium-high heat. Add the chicken breasts and sauté on both sides for about 6–7 minutes per side until golden brown. Remove the chicken from the skillet and place on a plate. Set aside.

3. Add the wine to the pan, scraping up any browned bits from the chicken. Reduce the wine until it almost evaporates. Add the remaining oil to the pan; add the onion and garlic and sauté for 5 minutes.

4. Puree the roasted red peppers with the milk and Italian seasoning. Add to the onion and garlic and cook for 1 minute. Add in the olives, capers, and sugar. Add back the chicken and nestle in the sauce, cook for 1 minute. Remove the pan from the heat and stir in the sour cream.

Exchanges/Choices

2 Vegetable	**Calories**	220	**Cholesterol**	70 mg	**Total Carbohydrate**	10 g
3 Lean Meat	Calories from Fat	70	**Sodium**	460 mg	Dietary Fiber	2 g
1/2 Fat	**Total Fat**	8.0 g	**Potassium**	375 mg	Sugars	6 g
	Saturated Fat	2.0 g			**Protein**	26 g
	Trans Fat	0.0 g			**Phosphorus**	215 mg

HERBS DE PROVENCE SEA BASS

Servings: 4   Serving Size: 4 ounces   Prep Time: 5 minutes   Cook Time: 15 minutes

One of the greatest joys of travel is a chance to sample the wonderful spices and herbs of each country I visit. When I long for my days in Provence, all I have to do is to open my stash of heady Herbs de Provence and I'm instantly transported to that sunny place. Herbs de Provence is a gentle blend, so I think it works well with fish dishes. The firm luscious flesh of sea bass with its buttery flavor pairs perfect with the lavender undertones of this herb blend.

1 pound	sea bass filets
1/2 teaspoon	Kosher salt
1/4 teaspoon	freshly ground black pepper
1 tablespoon	olive oil
1/2 teaspoon	unsalted butter
1/2 cup	diced onion
3	garlic cloves, minced
2 teaspoons	Herbs de Provence
1/3 cup	dry white wine
1/3 cup	low-fat, reduced-sodium chicken broth
1 teaspoon	coarse grain Dijon mustard

1. Sprinkle the sea bass with the salt and pepper. Heat the oil and butter in a large skillet over medium-high heat. Add the sea bass to the pan and sear on both sides for a total of 7–9 minutes until fish is cooked through. Remove the fish from the skillet, place on a plate, and set aside.

2. Add the onion and garlic to the pan and sauté for 5 minutes. Add in the Herbs de Provence and sauté 1 minute. Add in the wine and broth and boil over high heat, occasionally stirring until reduced to about 1/4 cup. Remove from the heat and whisk in the mustard. Drizzle a little sauce over each sea bass filet.

Exchanges/Choices

3 Lean Meat	**Calories**	165	**Cholesterol**	50 mg	**Total Carbohydrate**	4 g
1/2 Fat	Calories from Fat	55	**Sodium**	390 mg	Dietary Fiber	1 g
	Total Fat	6.0 g	**Potassium**	360 mg	Sugars	1 g
	Saturated Fat	1.4 g			**Protein**	22 g
	Trans Fat	0.0 g			**Phosphorus**	235 mg

GARLICKY SHRIMP

Servings: 6
Marinating time: 30 minutes
Serving Size: 2 ounces
Cook Time: 7 minutes
Prep Time: 5 minutes

It always amazes me that one ingredient could practically carry an entire dish. In this case the indispensable bulb of garlic is all you need to make tender shrimp shine. Just a tad of wine and pinch of red pepper flakes and you have what my niece calls an "awesome" meal!

5	garlic cloves, minced
1/4 teaspoon	dried red chili flakes
3 tablespoons	olive oil
12 ounces	uncooked frozen large shrimp, peeled and deveined, thawed and patted dry
1/2 cup	dry white wine
1/8 teaspoon	freshly ground black pepper

1. In a large bowl, combine the garlic, chili flakes, and oil and mix well. Add the shrimp and toss to coat. Cover the bowl and let the shrimp marinate in the refrigerator for 30 minutes.

2. Remove the shrimp from the refrigerator. Bring to room temperature.

3. Heat a large skillet over medium-high heat. Add the shrimp with the oil and sauté the shrimp for about 2 minutes per side. Remove the shrimp from the skillet.

4. Add the wine to the pan, scraping up any browned bits. Add the pepper. Bring to a boil and reduce to 1/4 cup. Pour the wine over the shrimp and serve.

Exchanges/Choices

2 Lean Meat	**Calories**	130	**Cholesterol**	90 mg	**Total Carbohydrate**	1 g
1 Fat	Calories from Fat	65	**Sodium**	480 mg	Dietary Fiber	0 g
	Total Fat	7.0 g	**Potassium**	130 mg	Sugars	0 g
	Saturated Fat	1.1 g			**Protein**	12 g
	Trans Fat	0.0 g			**Phosphorus**	130 mg

SCALLOP KEBABS

Servings: 4 **Serving Size:** 3 ounces **Prep Time:** 15 minutes **Cook Time:** 5–10 minutes

Here's a totally different way to prepare scallops. Most recipes will have you pan sear them, but why not try something new. I coat the scallops with crunchy panko crumbs seasoned with some Parmesan and garlic and thread them up into kebabs. Under the broiler, the outside gets crisp and the inside of the scallop stays silky.

8	wooden skewers
1/2 cup	panko breadcrumbs
2 tablespoons	grated fresh Parmesan cheese
3	garlic cloves, very finely minced, almost to a paste
1 teaspoon	Italian seasoning
12 ounces	large sea scallops, fresh or frozen, thawed and patted dry
	olive oil cooking spray

1. Add the wooden skewers to a pan of hot water. Set aside for 1–2 hours.

2. Cover a broiler pan with aluminum foil. Coat the foil with cooking spray. Preheat the oven broiler to high with the rack set about 5 inches from the heat source.

3. Combine the breadcrumbs, Parmesan cheese, garlic, and Italian seasoning together on a plate. Roll each scallop in the breadcrumb mixture.

4. Remove the wooden skewers from the hot water. Using two skewers per kebab, thread the scallops onto the skewers so the scallops are lying flat through the skewer.

5. Place the skewers on the prepared broiler pan. Coat each skewer with olive oil cooking spray. Broil the scallops for about 4 minutes per side until cooked through.

Exchanges/Choices

1/2 Starch	**Calories**	105	**Cholesterol**	25 mg	**Total Carbohydrate**	10 g
2 Lean Meat	Calories from Fat	15	**Sodium**	405 mg	Dietary Fiber	0 g
	Total Fat	1.5 g	**Potassium**	190 mg	Sugars	1 g
	Saturated Fat	0.6 g			**Protein**	13 g
	Trans Fat	0.0 g			**Phosphorus**	255 mg

CHICKEN THIGHS IN APRICOT PORT MUSTARD GLAZE

Servings: 4   Serving Size: 4 ounces   Prep Time: 15 minutes   Cook Time: 20 minutes

In feeding finicky tastes, I've always found that no one can resist a juicy chicken thigh coated with a good tangy sauce. With just three ingredients of apricot preserves, port, and mustard that combine to make a simple tasty sauce, no one will be finicky for long.

1 pound	boneless, skinless chicken thighs
1/2 teaspoon	Kosher salt
1/4 teaspoon	freshly ground black pepper
1 1/2 tablespoons	olive oil, divided
2	garlic cloves, minced
1/4 cup	no-sugar-added apricot preserves
1/4 cup	ruby port wine
2 teaspoons	Dijon mustard

1. Sprinkle the chicken with salt and pepper. Heat 1 tablespoon of olive oil in a large skillet over medium-high heat. Add the chicken thighs and sear on both sides for about 6–7 minutes per side. Remove the chicken from the skillet, add to a plate, and set aside.

2. Add the remaining oil to the pan and add the garlic. Sauté the garlic on medium heat for 1 minute. Mix together the preserves, port, and mustard and add to the garlic. Lower the heat and simmer for 2 minutes. Add back the chicken, nestle the chicken in the sauce, and cook on low heat for 1–2 minutes.

Exchanges/Choices

1/2 Carbohydrate	**Calories**	215	**Cholesterol**	105 mg	**Total Carbohydrate**	8 g
3 Lean Meat	Calories from Fat	100	**Sodium**	370 mg	Dietary Fiber	2 g
1 Fat	**Total Fat**	11.0 g	**Potassium**	255 mg	Sugars	2 g
	Saturated Fat	2.4 g			**Protein**	19 g
	Trans Fat	0.0 g			**Phosphorus**	175 mg

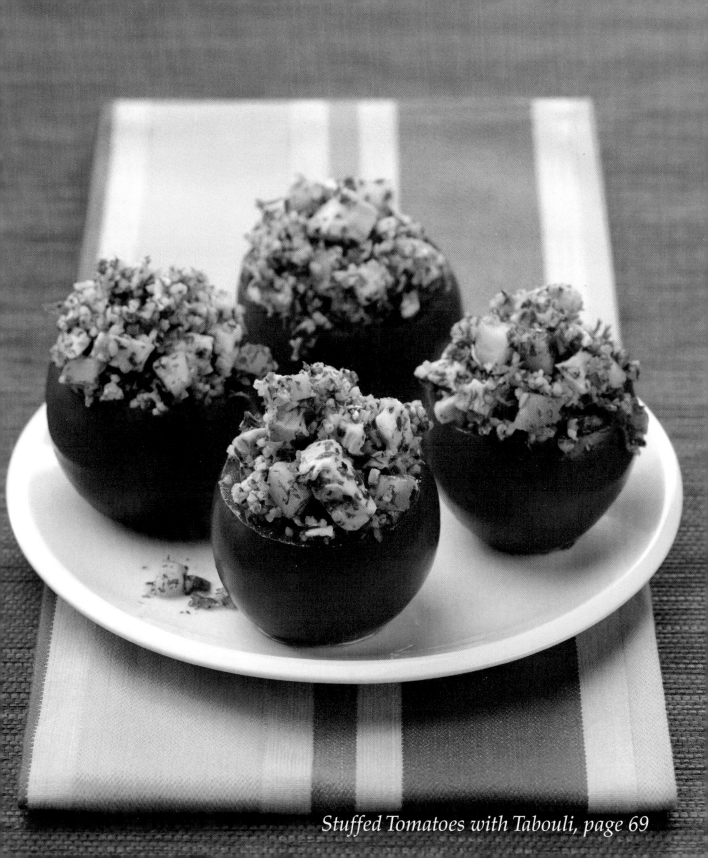

Stuffed Tomatoes with Tabouli, page 69

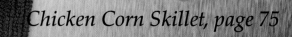

Chicken Corn Skillet, page 75

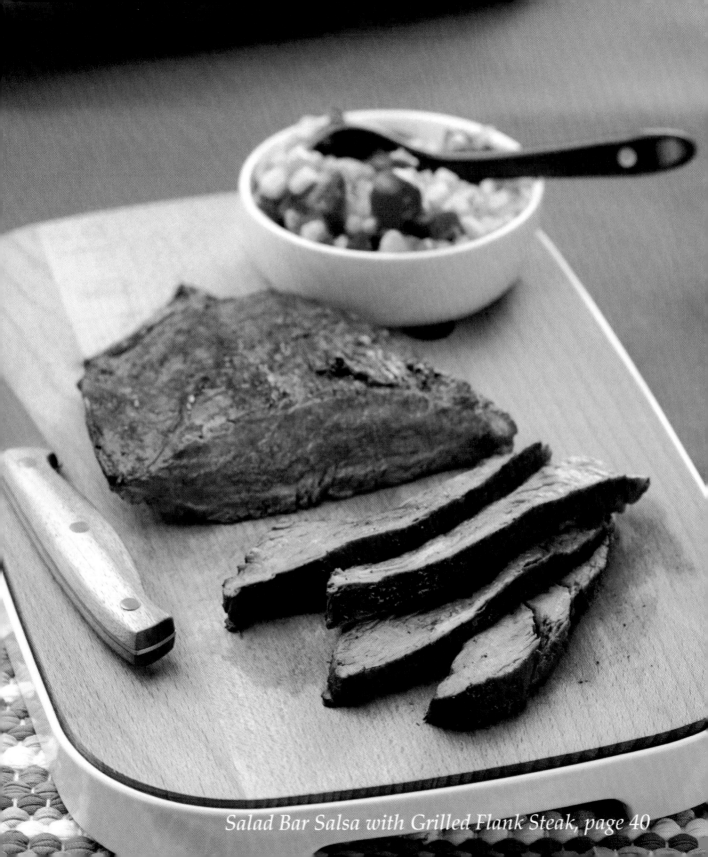

Salad Bar Salsa with Grilled Flank Steak, page 40

Chickpeas with Greens Soup, page 16; Fall Butternut Squash Soup, page 21; Tortilla Soup, page 23

Classic Spinach Pie, page 87

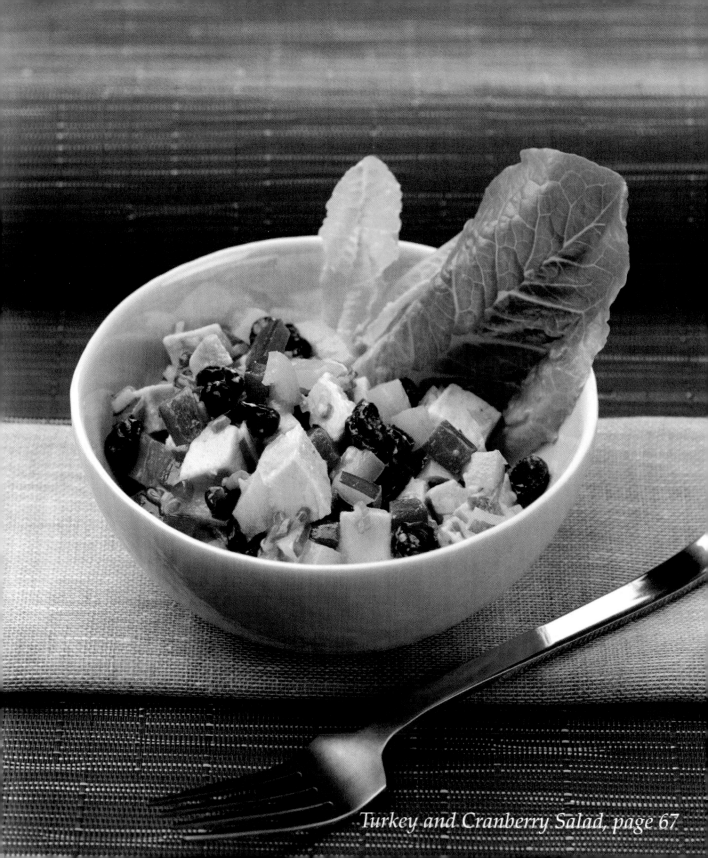

Turkey and Cranberry Salad, page 67

Chocolate Cherry Tarts, page 138; Grilled Balsamic Pineapple, page 144

Old Fashioned Ice Cream Soda, page 135

RIGATONI WITH SUN-DRIED TOMATOES, PESTO, AND OLIVES

Servings: 6   Serving Size: 3/4 cup   Prep Time: 15 minutes   Cook Time: 20 minutes

I'm always looking for new ways to serve large shapes of pasta. I've got the penne, fusilli, and shell shapes down pretty good, but I find shapes like rigatoni more of a challenge to balance with other ingredients. I've concluded that rigatoni just needs a few strong flavors such as olives, sun-dried tomatoes, and lemon zest to be special.

8 ounces	rigatoni (preferably whole-wheat)
	olive oil cooking spray
1/2 cup	diced onion
2	garlic cloves, minced
1/2 cup	sliced rehydrated sun-dried tomatoes (not packed in oil)
1/2 cup	dry white wine
4 tablespoons	bottled pesto sauce
2 tablespoons	toasted pine nuts
1/4 cup	pitted, coarsely chopped Kalamata olives
2 teaspoons	fresh lemon zest
	freshly ground black pepper to taste

1. Bring a large pot of lightly salted water to a boil. Add the rigatoni and cook for 8–10 minutes until al dente.

2. Meanwhile coat a large skillet with cooking spray. Sauté the onion and garlic over medium heat for about 6 minutes. Add the sun-dried tomatoes and sauté for 2 minutes. Add the wine and cook until wine is almost evaporated.

3. Drain the pasta, reserving about 1/3 cup pasta water. Set the pasta aside. Add the pasta water to the onion mixture and cook for 1 minute. Add in the pesto, pine nuts, olives, and lemon zest. Season with pepper. Add the rigatoni and toss well.

Exchanges/Choices

2 Starch	**Calories**	245	**Cholesterol**	0 mg	**Total Carbohydrate**	36 g
1 Vegetable	Calories from Fat	70	**Sodium**	235 mg	Dietary Fiber	5 g
1 1/2 Fat	**Total Fat**	8.0 g	**Potassium**	260 mg	Sugars	4 g
	Saturated Fat	1.0 g			**Protein**	7 g
	Trans Fat	0.0 g			**Phosphorus**	130 mg

ASIAN SESAME SHRIMP

Servings: 4
Marinating time: 30 minutes
Serving Size: 3 ounces
Cook Time: 6 minutes
Prep Time: 5 minutes

I love creating recipes that do double duty. These shrimp can be served as a main entree with a side of vegetables, or they can be skewered and served as a fun party appetizer. Also, try this marinade over chicken breasts.

Marinade

2 tablespoons	light soy sauce
2 tablespoons	rice vinegar
1 1/2 tablespoons	hoisin sauce
2 1/2 tablespoons	water
1 tablespoon	sesame seeds
1 teaspoon	sesame oil
2	garlic cloves, minced
1/2 teaspoon	hot mustard
1 pound	large fresh or frozen, thawed and patted dry, peeled and deveined uncooked shrimp

1. Combine all the ingredients for the marinade. Add the shrimp and toss to coat. Cover and refrigerate for 30 minutes.

2. Preheat the oven to 400 degrees. Remove the shrimp from the refrigerator and bring to room temperature. Line a broiler pan or baking sheet with foil. Coat the foil with cooking spray. Remove the shrimp from the marinade and pour the marinade into a small saucepan. Arrange the shrimp in a single layer on the prepared pan.

3. Roast the shrimp for about 6 minutes or until shrimp are cooked through and are opaque.

4. Boil the reserved marinade on medium-high heat for 1–2 minutes. Serve the sauce with the shrimp.

Exchanges/Choices

3 Lean Meat

Calories	145	**Cholesterol**	190 mg	**Total Carbohydrate**	4 g
Calories from Fat	25	**Sodium**	480 mg	Dietary Fiber	0 g
Total Fat	3.0 g	**Potassium**	300 mg	Sugars	2 g
Saturated Fat	0.4 g			**Protein**	25 g
Trans Fat	0.0 g			**Phosphorus**	265 mg

THAI TOFU

Servings: 4   Serving Size: 1 cup   Prep Time: 10 minutes   Cook Time: 25 minutes

When I first started eating tofu at home, all I knew how to do was to marinate it in soy sauce and then pan sear it. It was delicious, but after awhile I needed some new inspiration. The result is this recipe spiked with zesty red curry paste, garlic, and ginger and then cooled with coconut milk.

1 1/2 tablespoons	vegetable oil, divided
1 pound	extra firm tofu, drained and cut into 3/4-inch cubes
1/2 cup	sliced bell peppers (from the salad bar or produce section)
1/2 cup	cherry tomatoes (from the salad bar or produce section)
1/2 cup	sugar snap peas, trimmed
2	garlic cloves, minced
1 tablespoon	minced fresh ginger
2 tablespoons	bottled Thai red curry paste
1 cup	low-fat, reduced-sodium chicken or vegetable broth
1/2 cup	lite coconut milk

1. Heat 1 tablespoon of oil in a large skillet or wok over medium-high heat. Add the tofu, in batches if necessary, and cook until golden brown, about 5–6 minutes.

2. Remove the tofu with a slotted spoon and drain on paper toweling. Lower the heat to medium. Add the remaining oil to the pan. Add the bell peppers, tomatoes, and sugar snap peas and stir-fry for 3–4 minutes. Remove the vegetables from the pan. Add in the garlic and ginger and stir fry for 30 seconds. Add in the curry paste, then stir-fry for 30 seconds.

3. Add the broth and coconut milk to the pan and bring to a simmer. Simmer for 5 minutes. Add back the tofu and vegetables and simmer for 2 minutes. Serve over brown rice if desired.

Exchanges/Choices

1/2 Carbohydrate	**Calories**	180	**Cholesterol**	0 mg	**Total Carbohydrate**	9 g	
1 Med-Fat Meat	Calories from Fat	100	**Sodium**	445 mg	Dietary Fiber	2 g	
1 1/2 Fat	**Total Fat**	11.0 g	**Potassium**	345 mg	Sugars	3 g	
	Saturated Fat	2.5 g			**Protein**	11 g	
	Trans Fat	0.0 g			**Phosphorus**	170 mg	

LEMONY HERB CHICKEN

Servings: 5   Serving Size: 3 ounces   Prep Time: 5 minutes   Cook Time: 15–20 minutes

Citrus adds spark to any dish. All it takes to get a clean, fresh-tasting chicken dish is a lemon and a few aromatic herbs. Yes, dinner can be this simple.

Marinade

2 tablespoons	olive oil
2 tablespoons	fresh lemon juice
1 tablespoon	lemon zest
1 teaspoon	dried oregano
1 teaspoon	dried basil
1 teaspoon	dried thyme
1/4 teaspoon	crushed, dried chili flakes
1/4 teaspoon	Kosher salt
1/8 teaspoon	freshly ground black pepper
1 pound	boneless, skinless chicken thighs

1. Combine all the marinade ingredients in a large bowl. Add the chicken thighs and toss to coat. Cover and refrigerate for 3 hours or overnight.

2. Preheat the oven to 400 degrees. Cover a broiler pan with foil. Coat the foil with cooking spray. Drain the chicken from the marinade, discarding the marinade. Arrange the chicken in a single layer on the prepared pan.

3. Roast the chicken for about 15–20 minutes until the chicken reaches an internal temperature of 165 degrees.

Exchanges/Choices

2 Lean Meat						
1 Fat	**Calories**	145	**Cholesterol**	80 mg	**Total Carbohydrate**	1 g
	Calories from Fat	80	**Sodium**	145 mg	Dietary Fiber	0 g
	Total Fat	9.0 g	**Potassium**	180 mg	Sugars	0 g
	Saturated Fat	2.0 g			**Protein**	15 g
	Trans Fat	0.0 g			**Phosphorus**	135 mg

PORK LOIN CHOPS WITH MUSHROOM SAUCE

Servings: 4   **Serving Size:** 4 ounces   **Prep Time:** 15 minutes   **Cook Time:** 20 minutes

Do you serve seasonal dishes? We do in my house and when it's winter, hearty foods fit the bill. There is nothing more satisfying than woody mushrooms smothering lean seared pork chops on a cold wintry evening. I use the mushroom water as part of this fragrant sauce. Talk about resourceful!

1 ounce	packaged dried mushrooms (porcini, Portobello, shiitake)
3 tablespoons	flour
1/2 teaspoon	Kosher salt
1/4 teaspoon	freshly ground black pepper
1 1/2 tablespoons	olive oil
4 (4-ounce)	boneless pork loin chops, trimmed of excess fat
1/2 cup	diced onion
1/2 cup	dry white wine
2 tablespoons	tomato paste

1. Add the packaged mushrooms to a heatproof bowl. Add about 2/3 cup hot water to cover. Set aside for 15 minutes

2. Meanwhile, combine the flour, salt, and pepper. Dredge each pork chop in the flour mixture, shaking off the excess and discarding any unused flour. Drain the mushrooms, reserving the liquid. Coarsely chop the mushrooms.

3. Heat the olive oil over medium-high heat. Add the pork chops and sear on both sides for about 2–3 minutes per side. Remove the pork from the pan and set aside.

4. Add the onion to the skillet and sauté for about 5 minutes. Add in the mushrooms and sauté for 1 minute. Add in the reserved mushroom liquid. Mix together the white wine and tomato paste and add to the skillet. Bring to a boil, then lower the heat to simmer.

5. Add the pork chops to the skillet with any accumulated juice, nestling them in the sauce. Cook the pork chops for about 5 minutes on medium-low heat. Remove the pork chops from the pan and raise the heat to medium high. Boil the sauce just until the sauce thickens. Serve the sauce with the pork. Season with salt and pepper.

Exchanges/Choices

1 Carbohydrate	**Calories**	265	**Cholesterol**	60 mg	**Total Carbohydrate**	13 g
3 Lean Meat	Calories from Fat	110	**Sodium**	300 mg	Dietary Fiber	2 g
1 Fat	**Total Fat**	12.0 g	**Potassium**	535 mg	Sugars	2 g
	Saturated Fat	3.3 g			**Protein**	23 g
	Trans Fat	0.0 g			**Phosphorus**	215 mg

ROSEMARY TURKEY SALAD

| Servings: 4 | Serving Size: 1 cup | Prep Time: 10 minutes | Cook Time: 0 |

No-cook dishes are always a hit. Why slave over a hot stove, when you can serve this main dish turkey salad for lunch or dinner without "cooking". Try this with all kinds of other beans besides chickpeas and swap out the turkey for cooked chicken if you wish.

2 tablespoons	red wine vinegar
1 tablespoon	crumbled dried rosemary leaves
2	garlic cloves, minced
2 teaspoons	Dijon mustard
1/2 teaspoon	Kosher salt
1/8 teaspoon	freshly ground black pepper
2 tablespoons	olive oil
1 (15-ounce) can	chickpeas, drained and rinsed
2 cups	cubed (1/2-inch pieces) cooked turkey breast (from the deli)
1/2 cup	sliced celery (from the salad bar or produce section)
4 cups	greens (from the salad bar or produce section)

1. In a small bowl, whisk together the red wine vinegar, rosemary leaves, garlic, Dijon mustard, salt, and pepper. Slowly, in a thin stream, add the oil a little at a time whisking until emulsified.

2. Add the beans, turkey, and celery to the dressing and toss gently. Serve the salad over the greens.

Exchanges/Choices

1 Starch	**Calories**	275	**Cholesterol**	60 mg	**Total Carbohydrate**	20 g
4 Lean Meat	Calories from Fat	80	**Sodium**	470 mg	Dietary Fiber	6 g
1/2 Fat	**Total Fat**	9.0 g	**Potassium**	570 mg	Sugars	4 g
	Saturated Fat	1.4 g			**Protein**	28 g
	Trans Fat	0.0 g			**Phosphorus**	285 mg

LINGUINE WITH ARTICHOKES AND CAPERS

Servings: 6   Serving Size: 2/3 cup   Prep Time: 10 minutes   Cook Time: 10 minutes

I can never understand why we drown our pasta in so many ingredients. In Italy, pasta is served so simply that you wonder if there are any other ingredients in there besides the pasta. By using artichoke hearts, roasted red pepper, and capers, this dish goes way beyond the ubiquitous jarred sauce.

8 ounces	whole-wheat linguine (use low-carb versions, if desired)
6 ounces	marinated artichoke hearts, drained and quartered (reserve 1 tablespoon of the marinade)
1/4 cup	panko breadcrumbs
1 teaspoon	Italian seasoning
2 large	jarred roasted red peppers, drained, patted dry, and sliced
1 tablespoon	capers, drained

1. Bring a large pot of lightly salted water to a boil. Add the linguine and cook until al dente, about 6–7 minutes. Drain, reserving 1/3 cup of the pasta water. Return the pasta to the pot. Set aside.

2. Heat 1 tablespoon of reserved artichoke marinade in a medium skillet over medium heat. Add the panko breadcrumbs and Italian seasoning and cook the crumbs for about 2–3 minutes until golden brown.

3. Add the artichoke hearts, roasted red peppers, and capers to the pasta. Add in the reserved pasta cooking water and heat, tossing until slightly thickened, about 1–2 minutes.

4. Serve the pasta sprinkled with the panko breadcrumbs.

Exchanges/Choices

2 Starch

Calories	175	**Cholesterol**	0 mg	**Total Carbohydrate**	33 g
Calories from Fat	20	**Sodium**	215 mg	Dietary Fiber	5 g
Total Fat	2.0 g	**Potassium**	130 mg	Sugars	2 g
Saturated Fat	0.2 g			**Protein**	7 g
Trans Fat	0.0 g			**Phosphorus**	90 mg

SALMON CHICKPEA CAKES

Servings: 6   Serving Size: 2 cakes   Prep Time: 25 minutes   Cook Time: 8–10 minutes

Stuck for a brunch idea? Crispy salmon cakes that are bolstered with fiber-rich chickpeas make a perfect late morning meal. Try these cakes served with a crisp salad and spears of beautifully grilled fresh asparagus.

1 (14.75-ounce) can	red salmon, drained and any visible bones and skin removed, flaked with a fork
1 (15-ounce) can	chickpeas, drained and rinsed, partially mashed with a fork
1 cup	panko breadcrumbs
1	egg, beaten
1	egg white
1 teaspoon	hot sauce
1/2 teaspoon	ground cumin
1/4 teaspoon	Kosher salt
1/4 teaspoon	freshly ground black pepper
1 tablespoon	vegetable oil

1. Combine all ingredients except the oil in a large bowl and mix well. Form into cakes about 1/2-inch thick or less. Set the salmon chickpea cakes on a plate and place in the refrigerator for 30 minutes.

2. Remove the salmon chickpea cakes from the refrigerator. Heat the oil in a large skillet over medium-high heat. Add the cakes, in two batches, and cook for 4 minutes per side until golden brown.

Exchanges/Choices

1 1/2 Starch	**Calories**	235	**Cholesterol**	75 mg	**Total Carbohydrate**	20	g
2 Lean Meat	Calories from Fat	80	**Sodium**	425 mg	Dietary Fiber	3	g
1/2 Fat	**Total Fat**	9.0 g	**Potassium**	335 mg	Sugars	3	g
	Saturated Fat	1.4 g			**Protein**	20	g
	Trans Fat	0.0 g			**Phosphorus**	290	mg

THAI BROILED SHRIMP

Servings: 4   Serving Size: 4 ounces   Prep Time: 15 minutes   Cook Time: 10 minutes

If you like pepper, you will love this Thai-inspired shrimp dish. White peppercorns are not often used, but in my opinion they should be. These peppercorns are sharp in flavor but don't overwhelm. The toasting and grinding process of these peppercorns is a snap and the reward for your simple effort is a fresh, complex flavor.

1/2 tablespoon	white peppercorns
2 1/2 teaspoons	Asian fish sauce
1 teaspoon	sugar
1/8 teaspoon	crushed red chili flakes
1/8 teaspoon	Kosher salt
6	garlic cloves, minced
1 pound	extra large peeled and deveined uncooked shrimp, fresh or frozen and thawed

1. Add the peppercorns to a small skillet and toast over medium-high heat for 1 minute. Add the peppercorns to a spice grinder and process until ground.

2. Combine the ground peppercorns with the remaining ingredients in a bowl. Mix to coat the shrimp well. Cover and refrigerate for 30 minutes. Meanwhile cover a broiler pan with foil. Coat the foil with cooking spray, set aside.

3. Arrange the shrimp on the prepared pan and broil for about 6–7 minutes until shrimp are golden brown, turning once.

Exchanges/Choices

3 Lean Meat	**Calories**	115	**Cholesterol**	190 mg	**Total Carbohydrate**	4 g	
	Calories from Fat	0	**Sodium**	455 mg	Dietary Fiber	0 g	
	Total Fat	0.0 g	**Potassium**	305 mg	Sugars	1 g	
	Saturated Fat	0.1 g			**Protein**	25 g	
	Trans Fat	0.0 g			**Phosphorus**	245 mg	

PORK AU POIVRE

My first encounter with "au poivre" was with steak au poivre. Since I keep red meat to a minimum, this recipe is my experiment in using a very lean pork chop instead. Same magnificent flavor with some fat and calorie savings!

4 (4 ounces each)	very lean bone-in pork loin chops (about 1/2 inch thick)
1 tablespoon	coarsely ground black pepper
1 tablespoon	vegetable oil
1/2 cup	low-fat reduced-sodium chicken broth
1/2 cup	dry red wine
1 teaspoon	Dijon mustard
1 teaspoon	tomato paste
1/8 teaspoon	Kosher salt

1 Preheat the oven to 425 degrees. Line a baking sheet with parchment paper.

2 Sprinkle each side of the pork with the coarsely ground pepper. Heat the oil in a large oven proof skillet over medium high heat. Add the pork and sear for about 2 minutes per side. Add the pork to the prepared pan and roast in the oven for about 8–10 minutes.

3 Meanwhile, add the remaining ingredients to the skillet and heat on the stove over medium heat, stirring well with a whisk. Cook until reduced to about 1/2 cup. Remove the pork from the oven and serve the reduction over the pork.

Exchanges/Choices

3 Lean Meat	**Calories**	160	**Cholesterol**	45 mg	**Total Carbohydrate**	2 g
1/2 Fat	Calories from Fat	70	**Sodium**	200 mg	Dietary Fiber	1 g
	Total Fat	8.0 g	**Potassium**	280 mg	Sugars	1 g
	Saturated Fat	2.0 g			**Protein**	17 g
	Trans Fat	0.0 g			**Phosphorus**	110 mg

GINGER BLACK BEANS AND RICE

Servings: 4   Serving Size: 1 1/2 cups   Prep Time: 15 minutes   Cook Time: 7 minutes

The marriage of black beans and rice is a perfect match. Sometimes the combination can look a bit drab, but not here. Colorful bell peppers really perk up the color in this fabulous meatless meal. Try this dish with barley or quinoa if you have some leftover from another dish.

2 teaspoons	sesame oil
2	garlic cloves, minced
3	scallions, chopped
1 tablespoon	peeled, grated ginger
1 cup	diced red bell pepper
1 cup	diced yellow bell pepper
2 cups	black beans, drained and rinsed
2 cups	cooked brown rice (frozen brown rice or shelf-stable brown rice, heated through)

1   Heat the sesame oil in a large skillet or wok over medium heat. Add the garlic, scallions, and ginger and stir-fry for 30 seconds.

2   Add the peppers and stir fry for 3–4 minutes until peppers are soft. Add the black beans and simmer over medium-low heat until the beans are warmed though. Serve the black beans over brown rice.

Exchanges/Choices

2 1/2 Starch	**Calories**	250	**Cholesterol**	0 mg	**Total Carbohydrate**	46 g
1 Vegetable	Calories from Fat	30	**Sodium**	120 mg	Dietary Fiber	10 g
1/2 Fat	**Total Fat**	3.5 g	**Potassium**	540 mg	Sugars	5 g
	Saturated Fat	0.6 g			**Protein**	11 g
	Trans Fat	0.0 g			**Phosphorus**	215 mg

TUNA RICE CAKES

Servings: 4	Serving Size: 1 cake	Prep Time: 20 minutes	Cook Time: 10 minutes

My Mom was always inventive with a can of tuna. She could sure stretch this convenient fish into so many dishes. Here is one of my favorites from her old collection: still a real goodie!

2 cups	cooked brown rice (frozen and heated or shelf stable rice, heated)
1 (7-ounce) can	white meat tuna, drained and flaked
1/4 cup	plain breadcrumbs
1	egg, beaten
1 1/2 tablespoons	flour
1	garlic clove, minced
2 teaspoons	lite soy sauce
2 teaspoons	fresh minced chives
1/4 teaspoon	Kosher salt
1/4 teaspoon	freshly ground black pepper
1 tablespoon	canola oil

1. Combine the rice, tuna, breadcrumbs, egg, flour, garlic, soy sauce, chives, salt, and pepper. Mix well. Form into 4 cakes and place on a plate. Let the cakes rest for 15 minutes in the refrigerator.

2. Heat the canola oil in a large skillet over medium-high heat. Add the cakes and cook on each side for about 4–5 minutes per side or until golden brown. Drain on paper toweling.

Exchanges/Choices

2 Starch	**Calories**	235	**Cholesterol**	65 mg	**Total Carbohydrate**	27 g
2 Lean Meat	Calories from Fat	65	**Sodium**	465 mg	Dietary Fiber	2 g
	Total Fat	7.0 g	**Potassium**	180 mg	Sugars	1 g
	Saturated Fat	1.2 g			**Protein**	15 g
	Trans Fat	0.0 g			**Phosphorus**	205 mg

REFRIED BEAN PIZZAS

Servings: 4   Serving Size: 1 pizza   Prep Time: 20 minutes   Cook Time: 16 minutes

For a quick, healthy weekend lunch, these pizzas are a refreshing change from the usual sandwich. It's fun to prepare your own refried beans; all it takes is a little mashing and you've got a great individual pizza that's hearty and healthy.

1 tablespoon	olive oil
1 small	onion, chopped
2	garlic cloves, minced
1 (15-ounce) can	pinto beans, drained, rinsed, and coarsely mashed with a potato masher
2 teaspoons	mild or hot chili powder
1/2 teaspoon	ground cumin
1/4 teaspoon	oregano flakes
1 tablespoon	minced fresh cilantro
4 (8-inch)	whole-wheat tortillas
1/2 cup	reduced-fat shredded reduced-fat cheddar cheese
1/2 cup	diced tomatoes

1. Preheat the oven to 400 degrees. Heat the oil in a large skillet over medium heat. Add the onion and garlic and sauté for 3–4 minutes.

2. Add in the pinto beans, chili powder, cumin, and oregano and sauté for 1 minute.

3. Add in the beans. Raise the heat and mash the beans again, but not completely. Cook over high heat for 2 minutes.

4. Add in the cilantro and cook 1 minute. Place the tortillas on a large baking sheet. Spread the bean mixture evenly over the tortillas. Top with cheese and tomatoes. Bake for 6–9 minutes or until cheese melts and tortillas are crisp.

Exchanges/Choices

3 Starch	**Calories**	315	**Cholesterol**	5 mg	**Total Carbohydrate**	51 g
1 Lean Meat	Calories from Fat	65	**Sodium**	475 mg	Dietary Fiber	11 g
1/2 Fat	**Total Fat**	7.0 g	**Potassium**	545 mg	Sugars	2 g
	Saturated Fat	2.2 g			**Protein**	16 g
	Trans Fat	0.0 g			**Phosphorus**	295 mg

PESTO COUSCOUS AND CHICKPEAS

Servings: 4   Serving Size: 1 cup   Prep Time: 20 minutes
Cook Time: 12 minutes   Standing Time: 5 minutes

If you ask me what my favorite bottled condiment is, it would have to be pesto. While making your own pesto is not hard, nothing beats the ease of picking up a jar and adding a spoonful of the emerald green goodness into fluffy couscous. This main dish vegetarian meal will appeal to even the most diehard meat lover.

2 teaspoons	olive oil
1 small	onion, chopped
2 cloves	garlic, minced
1/2 cup	diced carrots
1/2 cup	diced zucchini
2 teaspoons	dried salt-free Italian seasoning
1 cup	whole-wheat couscous
2 cups	low-fat, reduced-sodium chicken broth
2 tablespoons	prepared pesto
1 (15-ounce) can	chickpeas, drained and rinsed

1. Heat the oil in a large skillet over medium heat. Add the onion and garlic and sauté for 3–4 minutes. Add the carrots and zucchini and sauté for 5 minutes.

2. Add in the Italian seasoning and sauté for 2 minutes. Add in the couscous and sauté for 1 minute. Add in the broth and bring to a boil. Cover and turn off the heat. Let the couscous stand covered for 5 minutes until the broth is absorbed.

3. Add in the pesto and chickpeas and mix gently.

Exchanges/Choices

3 Starch	**Calories**	335	**Cholesterol**	0 mg	**Total Carbohydrate**	56 g	
1 Vegetable	Calories from Fat	65	**Sodium**	420 mg	Dietary Fiber	10 g	
1 Lean Meat	**Total Fat**	7.0 g	**Potassium**	485 mg	Sugars	7 g	
1/2 Fat	Saturated Fat	1.0 g			**Protein**	14 g	
	Trans Fat	0.0 g			**Phosphorus**	230 mg	

ORANGE MARMALADE SALMON

Servings: 4   Serving Size: 4 ounces   Prep Time: 5 minutes   Cook Time: 10–12 minutes

Stocking a variety of sugar-free jams and preserves serves a purpose higher than just as a spread for toast. A sauce made from jewel-colored orange marmalade, tangy mustard, and aromatic spices can turn a simple piece of fish into something spectacular. Swap out the marmalade for apricot or peach preserves and watch the accolades roll in.

1/2 cup	sugar free orange marmalade
1 tablespoon	Dijon mustard
1/4 teaspoon	ground ginger
1/4 teaspoon	ground cumin
1/8 teaspoon	ground coriander
4 (4-ounce)	salmon filets

1. Preheat the oven to 400 degrees. Cover a broiler tray with foil. Coat the foil with cooking spray.

2. In a small bowl, combine the marmalade, mustard, ginger, cumin, and coriander.

3. Arrange the salmon filets on the broiler tray. Brush the filets with half of the marmalade mixture. Roast the salmon for about 6–7 minutes.

4. Turn the oven to broil. Brush the remaining marmalade mixture over the salmon and broil for about 4–5 minutes until the salmon is cooked through.

Exchanges/Choices

Exchanges/Choices							
1/2 Carbohydrate	**Calories**	225	**Cholesterol**	80 mg	**Total Carbohydrate**	11 g
3 Lean Meat	Calories from Fat	90	**Sodium**	150 mg	Dietary Fiber	4 g
1 Fat	**Total Fat**	10.0 g	**Potassium**	380 mg	Sugars	1 g
	Saturated Fat	1.8 g			**Protein**	25 g
	Trans Fat	0.0 g			**Phosphorus**	260 mg

CHAPTER 7
Quick & Easy Desserts

After a career of writing cookbooks for people with diabetes, I often hear from my dear readers how thankful they are that I include desserts in my books. For many of them, they are grateful for a simple piece of fruit turned into a special treat. Everyone, even if you have diabetes, needs a sweet finish to a meal every now and then. In this chapter, you'll find a new collection of sweet treats including tarts, cookies, puddings, grilled fruit, and more, that utilize the convenience of shelf-stable, frozen, and salad bar offerings.

Chocolate Cherry Tarts (pg 138) are sweet little gems that pair chocolate and juicy, plump cherries into a crisp, ready-made phyllo tart shell. Enjoy them anytime, but serving them for guests will certainly impress. Elevate a can of pineapple to new heights with *Grilled Balsamic Pineapple* (pg 144). Rich and intensely flavored balsamic vinegar caramelizes the pineapple when you add a smoky touch by quickly grilling pineapple rings. *Melon Coolers* (pg 147) are made with salad bar honeydew melon chunks that puree to a pretty emerald green, a deliciously satisfying end to a summer meal.

As you plan your meals, these desserts can also work as snacks if your food plan allows. As always, ask for assistance from a registered dietitian to assist in meal planning. After all, a little sweet pleasure is the spice of life!

PEACH AND BLUEBERRY SAUCE

Servings: 6 **Serving Size:** 1/4 cup **Prep Time:** 5 minutes **Cook Time:** 5-6 minutes

I love creating sauces to dress up yogurt, low-fat ice cream, or low-fat baked goods. You never have to worry about what time of year it is as peaches and blueberries are available anytime from your handy supermarket freezer section.

1 tablespoon	cornstarch or arrowroot
1/2 cup	fresh orange juice, divided
1/2 cup	water
1 1/2 tablespoons	light agave syrup
1/2 teaspoon	ground cinnamon
1/8 teaspoon	ground allspice
2 cups	frozen sliced peaches, thawed, drained, and cut into smaller pieces, if necessary
1/2 cup	frozen blueberries, thawed and drained
	Non-fat plain Greek yogurt

1 Combine the cornstarch with 3 tablespoons of the orange juice and mix well.

2 Add the cornstarch mixture, remaining orange juice, water, agave syrup, cinnamon, and allspice in a small saucepan and bring to a boil. Lower the heat and simmer until the sauce thickens.

3 Stir in the peaches and blueberries. Serve the sauce warm or cool to room temperature. Serve over Greek yogurt.

Exchanges/Choices

1 Carbohydrate							
Calories	60	**Cholesterol**	0 mg	**Total Carbohydrate**	15 g
Calories from Fat	0	**Sodium**	0 mg	Dietary Fiber	1 g
Total Fat	0.0 g	**Potassium**	160 mg	Sugars	11 g
Saturated Fat	0.0 g			**Protein**	1 g
Trans Fat	0.0 g			**Phosphorus**	15 mg

OLD FASHIONED ICE CREAM SODA

Serving: 1   **Serving Size:** 1 cup   **Prep Time:** 5 minutes

As a native New Yorker, one of the things we loved to sip on was a good old-fashioned ice cream soda. Here's a healthier version of that classic, prepared with just three ingredients you should always have on hand.

1 tablespoon	sugar free cocoa mix
1 cup	club soda
1/3 cup	low-fat ice cream such as Breyers 1/2 the fat Creamy Chocolate

1 Add the cocoa mix to a tall glass. Pour in about 3 tablespoons of the club soda and mix. Pour over the remaining club soda. Top with the ice cream. Add a little extra sweetener such as Splenda, if desired.

Exchanges/Choices

1 Carbohydrate

Calories	60	**Cholesterol**	5 mg	**Total Carbohydrate**	13 g
Calories from Fat	10	**Sodium**	100 mg	Dietary Fiber	2 g
Total Fat	1.0 g	**Potassium**	135 mg	Sugars	9 g
Saturated Fat	0.6 g			**Protein**	2 g
Trans Fat	0.0 g			**Phosphorus**	60 mg

PEANUT BUTTER COOKIE SANDWICHES

Servings: 8   **Serving Size:** 1 sandwich   **Prep Time:** 15 minutes

I must admit that the frosting of a cake has always been much more appealing to me than the cake itself. But gobs of frosting don't exactly fit into a healthy lifestyle, so how about just a small portion of it? With this simple homemade frosting spread between two peanut butter cookies, you can have creamy frosting in just the right amount.

1/2 cup	dark cocoa mix
1 tablespoon	confectioners' sugar
3 1/2 teaspoons	hot water
16	sugar-free peanut butter cookies, such as Murrays' Sugar Free

1. Mix together the cocoa mix, confectioners' sugar, and water and mix until smooth, adding more water if necessary. The texture should be like frosting.

2. Spread the cocoa mixture on one side of a peanut butter cookie. Top with another cookie to form a sandwich and press together. Repeat for all sandwiches.

Exchanges/Choices

1 Carbohydrate	**Calories**	115	**Cholesterol**	0 mg	**Total Carbohydrate**	15 g
1 Fat	Calories from Fat	65	**Sodium**	90 mg	Dietary Fiber	2 g
	Total Fat	7.0 g	**Potassium**	120 mg	Sugars	1 g
	Saturated Fat	2.0 g			**Protein**	3 g
	Trans Fat	0.1 g			**Phosphorus**	75 mg

APRICOT SMOOTHIE

Servings: 3   Serving Size: 2/3 cup   Prep Time: 5 minutes   Cook Time: 0

Sure, a smoothie can be dessert! This creamy drink will top off a meal in a most satisfying way. Move over milkshake, this smoothie has it all!

10–12	pitted canned apricot halves, packed in their own juice or water, drained
1 cup	fat-free milk or unsweetened almond milk
1/2 cup	sugar-free frozen vanilla yogurt
	dash almond extract

1. Combine all ingredients in a blender until smooth. Taste and adjust the sweetness level by adding a bit of Splenda, if necessary. Refrigerate the smoothies for 1/2 hour prior to serving. Serve in glasses.

Exchanges/Choices

1 1/2 Carbohydrate

Calories	115	**Cholesterol**	5 mg	**Total Carbohydrate**	26 g
Calories from Fat	0	**Sodium**	60 mg	Dietary Fiber	2 g
Total Fat	0.0 g	**Potassium**	315 mg	Sugars	20 g
Saturated Fat	0.1 g			**Protein**	5 g
Trans Fat	0.0 g			**Phosphorus**	125 mg

CHOCOLATE CHERRY TARTS

My husband's absolute favorite flavor combination is chocolate and cherry. Rich, sinful cocoa flavor paired with juicy, ripe cherries makes you feel like you really indulged. And with the ultimate convenience of frozen phyllo tart shells, these are perfect for entertaining and impressing guests.

16	frozen mini phyllo tart shells
1 package	sugar-free instant chocolate pudding, prepared according to package directions
2/3 cup	frozen pitted cherries, thawed, drained well, and chopped
1 cup	frozen sugar-free whipped topping
1/4 cup	toasted chopped unsalted peanuts

1. Preheat the oven to 375 degrees. Arrange the phyllo tarts on a large baking sheet. Bake the tarts for about 3–4 minutes just until warmed through. Remove the tarts from the oven.

2. Prepare the pudding, set aside one cup of the prepared pudding for another use. Fold the frozen thawed cherries into the remaining pudding.

3. Fill the tarts with cherry pudding mixture. Top each tart with whipped topping and sprinkle of peanuts.

Exchanges/Choices

1 Carbohydrate	**Calories**	100	**Cholesterol**	0 mg	**Total Carbohydrate**	11 g
1 Fat	Calories from Fat	55	**Sodium**	110 mg	Dietary Fiber	1 g
	Total Fat	6.0 g	**Potassium**	70 mg	Sugars	4 g
	Saturated Fat	1.4 g			**Protein**	2 g
	Trans Fat	0.0 g			**Phosphorus**	55 mg

TROPICAL PARFAITS

Servings: 6   **Serving Size:** 2/3 cup   **Prep Time:** 8 minutes   **Cook Time:** 20 minutes

One of the first desserts I learned to prepare was a parfait. The layering of ingredients I always find fun, yet it looks like you've worked all day to prepare. This one has some great exotic tropical flavors, yet with only 5 ingredients, you'll find yourself making this often.

1 (20-ounce) can	crushed pineapple in its own juice or water, undrained
1	banana, cut into small pieces
1/4 cup	fresh lime juice
2 cups	plain, non-fat Greek yogurt, stirred
1/4 cup	toasted shredded coconut

1 In a medium saucepan, combine the undrained pineapple, banana, and lime juice and bring to a simmer. Simmer on medium-low heat for 8–10 minutes until soft and lumpy. Remove the saucepan from the heat and add the sauce to a bowl. Cover and refrigerate for 1 hour.

2 In dessert dishes, layer the yogurt and sauce, ending with the sauce. Top each dessert dish with coconut.

Exchanges/Choices

1 Fruit	**Calories**	130	**Cholesterol**	0 mg	**Total Carbohydrate**	23 g
1/2 Fat-Free Milk	Calories from Fat	15	**Sodium**	45 mg	Dietary Fiber	2 g
1/2 Fat	**Total Fat**	1.5 g	**Potassium**	280 mg	Sugars	17 g
	Saturated Fat	1.3 g			**Protein**	8 g
	Trans Fat	0.0 g			**Phosphorus**	115 mg

GINGER PEAR COMPOTE

Servings: 3   Serving Size: 1/2 cup   Prep Time: 7 minutes   Cook Time: 5–6 minutes

Add some more fruit to any special occasions table. This compote is perfect for the winter holidays.

1 (20-ounce) can	pear halves, packed in their own juice or water, drained
1/4 cup	pear nectar
1	cinnamon stick
2	whole cloves
3 quarter-sized slices	crystallized ginger
1 tablespoon	lemon juice
Garnish	
	ground cinnamon

1. Chop the pears into small pieces. Add the pears, pear nectar, cinnamon stick, cloves, sliced ginger, and lemon juice to a medium saucepan. Bring to a gentle boil over medium-high heat.

2. Lower the heat and simmer on low for 6–7 minutes, until soft and aromatic. Remove the cinnamon sticks and cloves.

3. Add pears to dessert dishes and sprinkle with ground cinnamon.

Exchanges/Choices

1 1/2 Fruit						
Calories	80	**Cholesterol**	0 mg	**Total Carbohydrate**	21 g
Calories from Fat	0	**Sodium**	5 mg	Dietary Fiber	2 g
Total Fat	0.0 g	**Potassium**	115 mg	Sugars	15 g
Saturated Fat	0.0 g			**Protein**	0 g
Trans Fat	0.0 g			**Phosphorus**	15 mg

BLACKBERRY FOOL

Servings: 4   **Serving Size:** 1/2 cup   **Prep Time:** 5 minutes   **Cook Time:** 0

Fruit fools are an old fashioned creamy dessert, but I'm glad they are still around! Faster than preparing pudding, swirls of crimson colored blackberries make their way through rich sour cream and whipped cream. Decadence at its finest!

2 cups	frozen blackberries, thawed and drained
1/4 cup	Splenda sugar blend or brown sugar blend
1/2 cup	fat-free sour cream
1 cup	frozen fat-free whipped topping, thawed

Garnish

whole blackberries

1 Puree the blackberries with the Splenda. Add to a medium-sized bowl and fold in the sour cream and whipped topping gently, just until mixed and fluffy.

2 Serve in dessert dishes with additional whole blackberries for garnish.

Exchanges/Choices

1 1/2 Carbohydrate

Calories	100	**Cholesterol**	5 mg	**Total Carbohydrate**	22 g
Calories from Fat	5	**Sodium**	45 mg	Dietary Fiber	2 g
Total Fat	0.5 g	**Potassium**	100 mg	Sugars	11 g
Saturated Fat	0.2 g			**Protein**	2 g
Trans Fat	0.0 g			**Phosphorus**	50 mg

STRAWBERRY YOGURT CREAM

Servings: 8   Serving Size: 1/2 cup   Prep Time: 5 minutes

Who says you have to give up chocolate chips if you have diabetes? The highlight of this yogurt-based dessert is the fabulous little chocolate chips streaked throughout. Try this with frozen cherries also.

2 1/2 cups	fat-free Greek yogurt
1 1/3 tablespoons	honey
1 cup	frozen strawberries, thawed, drained well, and chopped into small pieces
3 tablespoons	mini chocolate chips
1/4 teaspoon	ground cinnamon

1   In a bowl, mix together the yogurt and honey until creamy. Fold in the strawberries, chocolate chips, and cinnamon. Serve in dessert dishes.

Exchanges/Choices

1 Carbohydrate
1/2 Fat

Calories	85	**Cholesterol**	0 mg	**Total Carbohydrate**	11 g
Calories from Fat	15	**Sodium**	30 mg	Dietary Fiber	0 g
Total Fat	1.5 g	**Potassium**	125 mg	Sugars	10 g
Saturated Fat	0.9 g			**Protein**	7 g
Trans Fat	0.0 g			**Phosphorus**	105 mg

CHOCOLATE BANANA PUDDING

Creamy silken tofu is my little secret to making this pudding smooth and rich. By freezing the bananas, you get a pudding so rich, you will think you're cheating on your healthy eating plan. You're not!

12 ounces	silken lite tofu
2 medium	peeled ripe bananas
1 tablespoon	Splenda brown sugar blend
3 tablespoons	mini chocolate chips, melted
1 teaspoon	pure vanilla extract
1/8 teaspoon	Kosher salt

1. In a blender, combine the tofu, bananas, and brown sugar and blend until smooth.

2. Add the melted chocolate, vanilla, and salt and blend until smooth. Pour the pudding into a bowl, cover, and refrigerate for 2 hours before serving.

For a thicker pudding, peel and freeze the bananas in a plastic bag overnight. Remove from the freezer and allow to stand at room temperature for 5 minutes. Break into chunks and add with the tofu and brown sugar and continue with the recipe.

Exchanges/Choices

1 1/2 Carbohydrate	**Calories**	155	**Cholesterol**	0 mg	**Total Carbohydrate**	25 g
1 Fat	Calories from Fat	35	**Sodium**	145 mg	Dietary Fiber	2 g
	Total Fat	4.0 g	**Potassium**	325 mg	Sugars	16 g
	Saturated Fat	2.0 g			**Protein**	6 g
	Trans Fat	0.0 g			**Phosphorus**	95 mg

GRILLED BALSAMIC PINEAPPLE

Servings: 4   **Serving Size:** 2 pineapple rings   **Prep Time:** 10 minutes   **Cook Time:** 3 minutes

There is nothing more decadent than caramelized pineapple. Grill pineapple with sweet honey and syrupy balsamic vinegar, and you've got a dessert that rivals any cake or pie.

2 tablespoons	good-quality balsamic vinegar (the thickest you can find)
8 slices	canned pineapple in its own juice, drained
1 tablespoon	honey
1 tablespoon	non-hydrogenated buttery spread, such as Smart Balance
1/4 cup	toasted almond slivers

1 Brush each pineapple slice with the vinegar.

2 Coat a grill pan with cooking spray. Add the pineapple slices and grill on both sides for about 2–3 minutes just until grill marks appear.

3 Heat the honey and buttery spread together in a microwave-safe container and microwave for 30 seconds.

4 Add the pineapple slices to individual serving dishes. Drizzle with the honey mixture. Top with the sliced almonds.

Exchanges/Choices

1/2 Fruit	**Calories**	125	**Cholesterol**	0 mg	**Total Carbohydrate**	18 g
1/2 Carbohydrate	Calories from Fat	55	**Sodium**	25 mg	Dietary Fiber	1 g
1 Fat	**Total Fat**	6.0 g	**Potassium**	150 mg	Sugars	16 g
	Saturated Fat	0.9 g			**Protein**	2 g
	Trans Fat	0.0 g			**Phosphorus**	40 mg

GINGERSNAP PEACHES

Even in the winter, I'll prepare a dessert with summer fruits. Canned peaches hold up well in baking. Here, I have infused a little holiday flavor with gingersnaps and pumpkin pie spice. You can also bake the whole thing in the oven instead of grilling.

3	gingersnap cookies, crushed
1 teaspoon	sugar
1/4 teaspoon	pumpkin pie spice
4	canned peach halves, in their own juice, drained
1 tablespoon	non-hydrogenated buttery spread, such as Smart Balance, melted

1. Heat an outdoor grill to medium heat. Tear off 4 (4 × 6-inch) squares of aluminum foil. Combine the cookies, sugar, and pumpkin pie spice.

2. Divide the peach halves among the foil squares. Stuff each peach cavity with the gingersnap mixture. Drizzle with the melted buttery spread. Fold the packages and crimp to seal.

3. Place the packages directly on the rack and heat for about 5 minutes. When ready to eat, carefully unwrap the foil and place the peach in a dessert dish.

Exchanges/Choices

1/2 Fruit	**Calories**	80	**Cholesterol**	0 mg	**Total Carbohydrate**	14 g
1/2 Carbohydrate	Calories from Fat	25	**Sodium**	60 mg	Dietary Fiber	1 g
1/2 Fat	**Total Fat**	3.0 g	**Potassium**	115 mg	Sugars	10 g
	Saturated Fat	0.8 g			**Protein**	1 g
	Trans Fat	0.0 g			**Phosphorus**	15 mg

CHOCOLATE DIPPED APRICOTS

Servings: 12   **Serving Size:** 2 whole apricots   **Prep Time:** 20 minutes   **Cook Time:** 2 minutes

Two ingredients are all it takes to add a sweet ending to any meal. Luscious plump dried apricots go for a chocolate dip; a fine finish that will impress.

2 ounces	semisweet chocolate
24	dried whole apricots

1. In a double boiler over simmering water, melt the chocolate.

2. Working quickly, dip one half of each apricot into the melted chocolate. Place the chocolate dipped apricots on a wire rack to dry before serving.

Exchanges/Choices

1 Carbohydrate

Calories	55	**Cholesterol**	0 mg	**Total Carbohydrate**	12 g
Calories from Fat	15	**Sodium**	0 mg	Dietary Fiber	1 g
Total Fat	1.5 g	**Potassium**	180 mg	Sugars	10 g
Saturated Fat	0.8 g			**Protein**	1 g
Trans Fat	0.0 g			**Phosphorus**	15 mg

MELON COOLERS

In the heat of summer, a simple dessert is the best. Skip the usual ice cream treats in favor of this healthy melon drink using convenient already cut fruit.

2 cups	honeydew or cantaloupe chunks (from the salad bar or cut fresh melons)
1/2 cup	orange juice
1 tablespoon	fresh lime juice
2 teaspoons	sugar
4	ice cubes
2	sprigs of fresh mint (optional)

1. Blend all the ingredients together in a blender and process for 30 seconds to 1 minute until smooth. Pour into tall glasses and serve. Garnish each glass with a sprig of fresh mint.

Exchanges/Choices

1 1/2 Fruit

Calories	100	**Cholesterol**	0 mg	**Total Carbohydrate**	24 g
Calories from Fat	0	**Sodium**	25 mg	Dietary Fiber	2 g
Total Fat	0.0 g	**Potassium**	555 mg	Sugars	22 g
Saturated Fat	0.1 g			**Protein**	2 g
Trans Fat	0.0 g			**Phosphorus**	35 mg

CINNAMON NACHOS WITH BLUEBERRY CREAM

Servings: 4
Prep Time: 20 minutes
Serving Size: 6 tortilla wedges, 1 1/2 ounces yogurt
Cook Time: 7–9 minutes

Who said nachos must be drowning in cheese? Packaged whole-wheat tortillas get transformed into a sweet treat when sprinkled with warm spices and topped with cool yogurt and fiber-rich blueberries.

3 (6-inch)	whole-wheat tortillas
	vegetable cooking spray
1 tablespoon	sugar
1/4 teaspoon	ground cinnamon
1/8 teaspoon	ground allspice
6 ounces	vanilla fat-free yogurt
1 cup	frozen blueberries, thawed and drained

1 Preheat the oven to 375 degrees. Cut each tortilla into 8 wedges. Place the wedges on a baking sheet. Coat the wedges with cooking spray. Combine the sugar, cinnamon, and allspice. Sprinkle the sugar mixture over the wedges. Bake for 7–9 minutes, until lightly browned. Remove the wedges from the oven and let cool.

2 Combine the yogurt and blueberries. For each serving, add 6 wedges to a dessert plate. Top with blueberry-yogurt mixture

Exchanges/Choices
1 1/2 Carbohydrate

Calories	110	**Cholesterol**	0 mg	**Total Carbohydrate**	23 g
Calories from Fat	10	**Sodium**	120 mg	Dietary Fiber	3 g
Total Fat	1.0 g	**Potassium**	130 mg	Sugars	9 g
Saturated Fat	0.2 g			**Protein**	3 g
Trans Fat	0.0 g			**Phosphorus**	85 mg

CHAPTER 8

Fast & Fabulous
Menu Planner

Day 1

1,500 Calories

Breakfast

Homemade zucchini pancakes:
  2 (4-inch) pancakes made with
  1/2 cup grated zucchini mixed
  in per serving, 2 tablespoons
  sugar-free syrup and
  1 tablespoon light margarine
  with sterols on top
1/2 cup unsweetened applesauce
1 oz Canadian bacon
1 cup skim milk

Calories	395
Calories from Fat	104
Total Fat	11.6 g
Saturated Fat	2.8 g
Trans Fat	0 g
Cholesterol	66 mg
Sodium	890 mg
Potassium	844 mg
Total Carbohydrate	65 g
Dietary Fiber	3 g
Sugars	26 g
Protein	21 g
Phosphorus	481 mg

Lunch

Lentil and Potato Stew (one
  serving)
2 small reduced fat whole wheat
  crackers
1/2 cup steamed green beans (no
  salt added) with 1 tablespoon
  light margarine with sterols
17 grapes
6 oz plain fat-free yogurt with
  1/8 cup low-fat granola and
  4 pecan halves dry mixed in
  (no salt)

Calories	524
Calories from Fat	101.7
Total Fat	11.3 g
Saturated Fat	2.8 g
Trans Fat	0.01 g
Cholesterol	3.4 mg
Sodium	699 mg
Potassium	1557 mg
Total Carbohydrate	80 g
Dietary Fiber	12 g
Sugars	39 g
Protein	24 g
Phosphorus	604 mg

Dinner

Roasted Shrimp with Cabbage
  Slaw (1 serving)*
2/3 cup couscous (no salt added)
raw vegetables from salad bar—
  1 cup broccoli and 1 cup carrots
  with 1 tablespoon reduced-fat
  ranch dressing
1 large fresh pear
8 pistachios (no added salt)

Calories	562
Calories from Fat	151
Total Fat	16.8 g
Saturated Fat	1.6 g
Trans Fat	0 g
Cholesterol	124 mg
Sodium	558 mg
Potassium	1181 mg
Total Carbohydrate	81 g
Dietary Fiber	16 g
Sugars	32 g
Protein	26 g
Phosphorus	364 mg

*Recipe included in book

DAY 1 total nutritional value

Calories	1480	**Cholesterol**	194 mg	**Total Carbohydrate**	226 g
Calories from Fat	357.3	**Sodium**	2146 mg	Dietary Fiber	31 g
Total Fat	39.7 g	**Potassium**	3581 mg	Sugars	96 g
Saturated Fat	7.2 g			**Protein**	62 g
Trans Fat	0.01 g			**Phosphorus**	1448 mg

Day 2
1,500 Calories

Breakfast

1 serving Hash Brown Quiche*
1 medium sliced tomato, 1 1/2 oz slice pumpernickel toast with 1/2 tablespoon light margarine with stanols
1 cup skim milk
1/2 cup orange juice

Calories	390
Calories from Fat	77
Total Fat	8.6 g
Saturated Fat	2.6 g
Trans Fat	0 g
Cholesterol	55 mg
Sodium	725 mg
Potassium	1234 mg
Total Carbohydrate	59 g
Dietary Fiber	7 g
Sugars	28 g
Protein	21 g
Phosphorus	482 mg

Lunch

Vegetable salad made with:
  1 1/2 cups raw spinach, 1/2 cup sliced cucumber, 1/2 cup red beets (canned low sodium), 1/2 cup broccoli, 1/2 cup green peppers, and 2 tablespoons Italian fat-free salad dressing
6 oz skim milk yogurt mixed with 2 oz banana + 1 small plum
2 oz multigrain with raisins bagel with 1 tablespoon almond butter without salt and 1 teaspoon light jam

Calories	535
Calories from Fat	103
Total Fat	11.5 g
Saturated Fat	1.3 g
Trans Fat	0 g
Cholesterol	4 mg
Sodium	770 mg
Potassium	2051 mg
Total Carbohydrate	91 g
Dietary Fiber	14 g
Sugars	48 g
Protein	25 g
Phosphorus	629 mg

Dinner

Italian Turkey Saute (1 serving)*
2/3 cup spinach pasta cooked without salt
Fruit cup made with 1 medium peach (6 oz) + 1 cup raspberries and 5 hazelnuts
1/2 cup Italian beans (low sodium) with 1/2 cup raw cranberries sweetened with sugar substitute,
8 large black olives

Calories	555
Calories from Fat	132
Total Fat	14.7 g
Saturated Fat	1.7 g
Trans Fat	0 g
Cholesterol	60 mg
Sodium	720 mg
Potassium	1344 mg
Total Carbohydrate	78 g
Dietary Fiber	18 g
Sugars	23 g
Protein	36 g
Phosphorus	450 mg

DAY 2 total nutritional value

Calories	1480	**Cholesterol**	119 mg	**Total Carbohydrate**	229 g
Calories from Fat	313.2	**Sodium**	2216 mg	Dietary Fiber	39 g
Total Fat	34.8 g	**Potassium**	4629 mg	Sugars	99 g
Saturated Fat	5.7 g			**Protein**	82 g
Trans Fat	0 g			**Phosphorus**	1562 mg

Day 3
1,500 Calories

Breakfast

4 oz oat bran with nuts muffin
   (2 teaspoon light jam,
   1 teaspoon light margarine with
   stanols on top)
3/4 cup blackberries
8 oz 1% milk
1/2 cup canned vegetable juice
   (low sodium)

Calories	362
Calories from Fat	80
Total Fat	8.8 g
Saturated Fat	2.7 g
Trans Fat	0 g
Cholesterol	12 mg
Sodium	442 mg
Potassium	1073 mg
Total Carbohydrate	60 g
Dietary Fiber	10 g
Sugars	31 g
Protein	15 g
Phosphorus	491 mg

Lunch

Salad Bar Roasted Vegetable
   Salad (one serving)*
1 oz grilled salmon
1 small 100% whole-wheat dinner
   roll
1 milkshake (blend 3 oz skim milk
   yogurt, 4 oz 1% milk 1 small
   [4 oz] banana, 3/4 teaspoon
   crunchy peanut butter, and
   1/2 cup shaved ice)

Calories	546
Calories from Fat	139.5
Total Fat	15.5 g
Saturated Fat	3.2 g
Trans Fat	0 g
Cholesterol	26 mg
Sodium	666 mg
Potassium	1646 mg
Total Carbohydrate	80 g
Dietary Fiber	12 g
Sugars	38 g
Protein	27 g
Phosphorus	571 mg

Dinner

Chicken in Blueberry Sauce
   (1 serving)*
1/3 cup long grain brown rice
   (no salt added in cooking)
   mixed with 1/2 cup wild rice (no
   added salt in cooking), 1/2 cup
   cucumbers, 1/2 cup peppers,
   4 pecan halves
1 cup steamed Brussels sprouts
   no-salt-added with 1 tablespoon
   light margarine with stenols
1/2 cup unsweetened applesauce

Calories	579
Calories from Fat	99
Total Fat	11 g
Saturated Fat	3.5 g
Trans Fat	0 g
Cholesterol	65 mg
Sodium	604 mg
Potassium	1195 mg
Total Carbohydrate	78 g
Dietary Fiber	11 g
Sugars	21 g
Protein	35 g
Phosphorus	447 mg

DAY 3 total nutritional value

Calories	1486	**Cholesterol**	103 mg	**Total Carbohydrate**	218 g
Calories from Fat	318.6	**Sodium**	1712 mg	Dietary Fiber	33 g
Total Fat	35.4 g	**Potassium**	3914 mg	Sugars	91 g
Saturated Fat	9.4 g			**Protein**	76 g
Trans Fat	0 g			**Phosphorus**	1510 mg

Day 4
1,500 Calories

Breakfast

(2 oz) 7 grain bread (toasted)
with 1 tablespoon light
margarine with stanols
Fruit salad made with 6 raw
cherries + 2 oz pear
1/4 cup cottage cheese (1% fat,
no sodium added) mixed with
2 teaspoon light jam
1 cup skim milk

Calories	405
Calories from Fat	75
Total Fat	8.3 g
Saturated Fat	2.5 g
Trans Fat	0 g
Cholesterol	7 mg
Sodium	429 mg
Potassium	749 mg
Total Carbohydrate	59 g
Dietary Fiber	7 g
Sugars	34 g
Protein	24 g
Phosphorus	471 mg

Lunch

1 serving Aromatic Indian Style
Pea Soup (with 2 leaves fresh
spearmint sprigs)*
1.5 oz Naan with 1 1/2 tablespoons
light margarine with stanols
6 oz plain non-fat yogurt with
1 cup cucumbers
1 cup cubed papaya

Calories	482
Calories from Fat	140
Total Fat	15.6 g
Saturated Fat	5.8 g
Trans Fat	0 g
Cholesterol	16 mg
Sodium	870 mg
Potassium	1325 mg
Total Carbohydrate	64 g
Dietary Fiber	7 g
Sugars	30 g
Protein	21 g
Phosphorus	449 mg

Dinner

Barbequed Chicken Sandwiches
(1 serving)*
Fruit salad made with 3/4 cup
honeydew melon + 3/4 cup
cantaloupe cubes
Coleslaw made with: 1/2 cup
shredded raw carrots +
1/2 cup shredded raw cabbage
and 1 tablespoon reduced
fat mayonnaise + vinegar
1 tablespoon
3/4 cup steamed green beans
(no added salt) + 1/4 cup water
chestnuts and 1 tablespoon light
margarine with stanols

Calories	582
Calories from Fat	142
Total Fat	15.8 g
Saturated Fat	3.5 g
Trans Fat	0.02 g
Cholesterol	65 mg
Sodium	752 mg
Potassium	1820 mg
Total Carbohydrate	86 g
Dietary Fiber	13 g
Sugars	48 g
Protein	30 g
Phosphorus	418 mg

DAY 4 total nutritional value

Calories	1468	**Cholesterol**	89 mg	**Total Carbohydrate**	209 g	
Calories from Fat	358.2	**Sodium**	2052 mg	Dietary Fiber	28 g	
Total Fat	39.8	**Potassium**	3895 mg	Sugars	111 g	
Saturated Fat	11.8 g			**Protein**	75 g	
Trans Fat	0.016 g			**Phosphorus**	1338 mg	

Day 5

1,500 Calories

Breakfast

2 servings Classic Spinach Pie*
3/4 cup sectioned grapefruit with
   1/4 cup blueberries
8 oz 1% milk
1/2 cup low sodium tomato juice

Calories	399
Calories from Fat	78
Total Fat	8.7 g
Saturated Fat	3.6 g
Trans Fat	0 g
Cholesterol	52 mg
Sodium	520 mg
Potassium	1252 mg
Total Carbohydrate	69 g
Dietary Fiber	7 g
Sugars	35 g
Protein	18.5 g
Phosphorus	402 mg

Lunch

1 (10-inch) whole-wheat tortilla
   roll made with 1/3 cup fresh
   Mung bean sprouts, 1/3 cup
   shredded napa cabbage,
   1/3 cup shredded carrots,
   1 oz turkey pastrami, 2 oz
   avocado, and 1 tablespoon
   fat-free honey mustard
1/2 cup steamed broccoli spears
   (no added salt)
6 oz non-fat yogurt mixed with
   4 fresh apricots (total
   5 1/2 oz apricots)
1 cup light popcorn (no salt)

Calories	577
Calories from Fat	111
Total Fat	12.3 g
Saturated Fat	2.1 g
Trans Fat	0 g
Cholesterol	23 mg
Sodium	1012 mg
Potassium	1777 mg
Total Carbohydrate	95 g
Dietary Fiber	17 g
Sugars	35 g
Protein	30 g
Phosphorus	567 mg

Dinner

Pork Au Poivre (1 serving)*
2/3 cup long grain brown rice
   (no added salt)
3/4 cup canned beets
3/4 cup cooked spinach (boiled,
   drained no salt) with
   1 1/2 tablespoons light
   margarine with stanols
1 small fresh orange mixed with
   1 kiwi and 2 tablespoons light
   whipped topping

Calories	513
Calories from Fat	169
Total Fat	18.8 g
Saturated Fat	5.6 g
Trans Fat	0 g
Cholesterol	45 mg
Sodium	658 mg
Potassium	1385 mg
Total Carbohydrate	58 g
Dietary Fiber	11 g
Sugars	18 g
Protein	27 g
Phosphorus	345 mg

DAY 5 total nutritional value

Calories	1503	**Cholesterol**	120 mg	**Total Carbohydrate**	225 g
Calories from Fat	358	**Sodium**	2212 mg	Dietary Fiber	36 g
Total Fat	39.8 g	**Potassium**	4518 mg	Sugars	89 g
Saturated Fat	11.4 g			**Protein**	75 g
Trans Fat	0 g			**Phosphorus**	1407 mg

Day 1
1,800 Calories

Breakfast

2 oz Rye toast with 1 tablespoon light margarine with plant sterols and 2 teaspoons light jam
1 cup fresh raspberries mixed with 1 cup honeydew melon
1 cup steamed 1% milk, mix with 1/2 teaspoon vanilla extract, and 1-2 shots espresso, add sugar substitute if desired, add 2 tablespoons light whipped topping (steamed latte)
Egg white omelet with 1/4 cup egg substitute (plain), 1/2 cup mixed mushrooms and zucchini (cooked total amount, use cooking spray to spray pan) may use salt-free seasoning blends on omelet if desired.

Calories	556
Calories from Fat	130
Total Fat	14.5 g
Saturated Fat	4.4 g
Trans Fat	0 g
Cholesterol	14.1 mg
Sodium	761 mg
Potassium	1588 mg
Total Carbohydrate	83 g
Dietary Fiber	14 g
Sugars	42 g
Protein	25 g
Phosphorus	512 mg

Lunch

One serving Turkey and Cranberry Salad*
2 small 100% whole-wheat rolls
1 cup green beans cooked with 1/2 tsp olive oil
1 large pear cut up with 6 oz skim milk yogurt

Calories	647
Calories from Fat	153
Total Fat	17 g
Saturated Fat	2.6 g
Trans Fat	0 g
Cholesterol	33 mg
Sodium	850 mg
Potassium	1554 mg
Total Carbohydrate	97 g
Dietary Fiber	18 g
Sugars	50 g
Protein	34 g
Phosphorus	650 mg

Dinner

Scallop Kebabs*
3/4 cup cooked wild rice (no added salt)
2 slices low-sodium wheat crisp bread
1/2 cup roasted beets mixed with 1 cup escarole**
1/2 cup steamed asparagus with 1 tablespoon light margarine with plant sterols
1 small orange
1/2 cup apple juice mixed with 1 cup seltzer water over shaved ice.

**To roast beets—heat oven to 400 degrees. Wash beets thoroughly, place beets on a sheet of tin foil placed on a baking tray. Drizzle 1.5 teaspoons canola oil for each serving over the top. Wrap the tin foil around the beets and roast until tender (30–50 minutes; a knife or fork should easily pierce the beet when done), let cool and peel. Cut in bite-sized pieces and mix with washed escarole.

Calories	572
Calories from Fat	129
Total Fat	14.4 g
Saturated Fat	2.7 g
Trans Fat	0 g
Cholesterol	25 mg
Sodium	614 mg
Potassium	1162 mg
Total Carbohydrate	88 g
Dietary Fiber	8 g
Sugars	26 g
Protein	23 g
Phosphorus	469 mg

DAY 1 total nutritional value

Calories	1776	**Cholesterol**	72 mg	**Total Carbohydrate**	269 g
Calories from Fat	413	**Sodium**	2226 mg	Dietary Fiber	42 g
Total Fat	45.9 g	**Potassium**	4314 mg	Sugars	119 g
Saturated Fat	9.9 g			**Protein**	84 g
Trans Fat	0 g			**Phosphorus**	1631 mg

Day 2
1,800 Calories

Breakfast

Whole-wheat English muffin (full muffin) with 1 medium tomato and 1 oz low-sodium Swiss cheese**

Blackberry kiwi smoothie (blend 1 cup skim milk, 3/4 cup black berries, 1 kiwi, and ice in blender)

**(Toast English muffin. In small pan heat margarine and pan fry tomato slices. Stack tomato slices on English muffin halves. Put 1/2 oz of cheese on top of the tomato and heat in microwave until cheese is melted.)

Calories	440
Calories from Fat	115
Total Fat	12.8 g
Saturated Fat	6.2 g
Trans Fat	0 g
Cholesterol	31 mg
Sodium	502 mg
Potassium	1231 mg
Total Carbohydrate	62 g
Dietary Fiber	13 g
Sugars	33 g
Protein	25 g
Phosphorus	652 mg

Lunch

1 serving Mushroom Polenta*
1 slice Italian bread (1 oz)
2 medium fresh figs
1/2 cup steamed broccoli (no added fat or salt)
2 oz roasted chicken (no skin)
100% frozen juice bar

Calories	761
Calories from Fat	146
Total Fat	16.2 g
Saturated Fat	4.5 g
Trans Fat	0.1 g
Cholesterol	65 mg
Sodium	806 mg
Potassium	1802 mg
Total Carbohydrate	116 g
Dietary Fiber	14 g
Sugars	59 g
Protein	42 g
Phosphorus	630 mg

Dinner

1 serving Beans and Greens with Whole-Wheat Shells*
100% whole-wheat roll (1 oz)
1 1/4 cup cut strawberries + 3/4 cup cut blueberries fruit cup
Salad**

**(1 cup romaine lettuce, 1/2 cup cucumbers, 4 medium baby carrots, 5 cherry tomatoes, 1/2 cup chopped green pepper, 1/2 cup raw pea pods, dressing made with 1 teaspoon olive oil and 1/8 cup red wine vinegar + 1 oz tuna [canned in water and drained) mixed with 1 teaspoon mayonnaise.]

Calories	575
Calories from Fat	95
Total Fat	10.5 g
Saturated Fat	2.7 g
Trans Fat	0 g
Cholesterol	12 mg
Sodium	480 mg
Potassium	1457 mg
Total Carbohydrate	93 g
Dietary Fiber	19 g
Sugars	34 g
Protein	23 g
Phosphorus	411 mg

DAY 2 total nutritional value

Calories	1775	**Cholesterol**	108.6 mg	**Total Carbohydrate**	271.2 g
Calories from Fat	354.6	**Sodium**	1788 mg	Dietary Fiber	45.8 g
Total Fat	39.4 g	**Potassium**	4491 mg	Sugars	125.4 g
Saturated Fat	13.4 g			**Protein**	90 g
Trans Fat	0.1 g			**Phosphorus**	1693 mg

Day 3
1,800 Calories

Breakfast

2 slices raisin bread toast with
  1 tablespoon light margarine
  with sterols and 2 teaspoons
  light jam
1/4 cup cottage cheese
  (1% no sodium added)
1 cup mango
1 cup skim milk

Calories	458
Calories from Fat	84
Total Fat	9.1 g
Saturated Fat	2.8 g
Trans Fat	0 g
Cholesterol	7 mg
Sodium	432 mg
Potassium	859 mg
Total Carbohydrate	75 g
Dietary Fiber	5 g
Sugars	44 g
Protein	22 g
Phosphorus	415 mg

Lunch

2 oz broiled turkey Patty
  (93% lean) on a 100% whole
  wheat hamburger bun (2 oz)
  with 1 leaf of lettuce and one
  slice tomato, 1 tablespoon low
  sodium ketchup, 1 teaspoon
  mustard
One serving Mixed Mushroom
  Soup*
1/2 cup mixed cooked corn + peas
  (from frozen)
24 fresh sweet Bing cherries
6 oil-roasted cashews without salt
1 cup 1% milk

Calories	681
Calories from Fat	179
Total Fat	19.9 g
Saturated Fat	5.9 g
Trans Fat	0.1 g
Cholesterol	72 mg
Sodium	720 mg
Potassium	1735 mg
Total Carbohydrate	97 g
Dietary Fiber	12 g
Sugars	52 g
Protein	37 g
Phosphorus	687 mg

Dinner

Grilled veggies and fish**
Ginger Pear Compote*

** In grill basket place the
  following foods and grill: 5 oz
  corn-on the cob, 6 oz baked
  sweet potato, 1 cup raw
  cabbage, 1/2 cup raw green
  pepper, 1/2 cup raw zucchini,
  1/2 cup raw mushrooms,
  1/2 cup raw tomato, 2 oz grilled
  sea bass or mahi-mahi,
  1/4 cup canned pineapple.
  2 tablespoons light margarine
  containing omega, and
  1 tablespoon fat-free sour cream
  on top of vegetables and fish
  after cooked.

Calories	625
Calories from Fat	127
Total Fat	14.1 g
Saturated Fat	5.2 g
Trans Fat	0 g
Cholesterol	31 mg
Sodium	600 mg
Potassium	2333 mg
Total Carbohydrate	106 g
Dietary Fiber	17 g
Sugars	44 g
Protein	26 g
Phosphorus	498 mg

DAY 3 total nutritional value

Calories	1765	**Cholesterol**	110 mg	**Total Carbohydrate**	278 g
Calories from Fat	389	**Sodium**	1753 mg	Dietary Fiber	35 g
Total Fat	43.2 g	**Potassium**	4927 mg	Sugars	140 g
Saturated Fat	14 g			**Protein**	85 g
Trans Fat	0.018 g			**Phosphorus**	1600 mg

Day 4
1,800 Calories

Breakfast

1 cup prepared instant oatmeal (low sodium) with 1 medium peach (6 oz) cut up
6 oz plain non-fat yogurt mixed with 4 English walnut halves and 3 prunes

Calories	493
Calories from Fat	91
Total Fat	10.1 g
Saturated Fat	1.5 g
Trans Fat	0 g
Cholesterol	3 mg
Sodium	295 mg
Potassium	1214 mg
Total Carbohydrate	87 g
Dietary Fiber	10 g
Sugars	38 g
Protein	21 g
Phosphorus	607 mg

Lunch

One Roast Beef Roll Up*
8 potato chips without salt and reduced fat
1 cup cooked carrots (no salt added) with 1 tablespoon light margarine with plant sterols
1 1/4 cups watermelon cubes
1 small unfrosted brownie (1 oz)
1 cup skim milk

Calories	698
Calories from Fat	106
Total Fat	11.8 g
Saturated Fat	4.7 g
Trans Fat	0 g
Cholesterol	45 mg
Sodium	913 mg
Potassium	1675 mg
Total Carbohydrate	107 g
Dietary Fiber	13 g
Sugars	43 g
Protein	32 g
Phosphorus	632 mg

Dinner

1 serving Orange Marmalade Salmon*
5/6 cup cooked quinoa
4 oz sliced apples with skin+ 3/4 cup wild Alaskan blueberries
1 1/2 cup steamed spinach (no salt added) with 1 tablespoon light margarine with plant sterols

Calories	626
Calories from Fat	175
Total Fat	19.4 g
Saturated Fat	3.5 g
Trans Fat	0 g
Cholesterol	80 mg
Sodium	435 mg
Potassium	2079 mg
Total Carbohydrate	79 g
Dietary Fiber	19 g
Sugars	19 g
Protein	41 g
Phosphorus	689 mg

DAY 4 total nutritional value

Calories	1817	**Cholesterol**	128 mg	**Total Carbohydrate**	273 g
Calories from Fat	372	**Sodium**	1644 mg	Dietary Fiber	43.3 g
Total Fat	41.3 g	**Potassium**	4968 mg	Sugars	100 g
Saturated Fat	9.6 g			**Protein**	94 g
Trans Fat	0 g			**Phosphorus**	1928 mg

Day 5
1,800 Calories

Breakfast

1 cup yellow corn grits (enriched, prepared without salt) and mix in 1 oz low-fat cheddar cheese
1 cup honeydew melon balls mixed with 1 1/4 cup strawberries and 1 tablespoon pine nuts
1 cup skim milk

Calories	461.6
Calories from Fat	87
Total Fat	9.62 g
Saturated Fat	2 g
Trans Fat	0 g
Cholesterol	10.9 mg
Sodium	314.9 mg
Potassium	1181 mg
Total Carbohydrate	76 g
Dietary Fiber	7 g
Sugars	36 g
Protein	21.3 g
Phosphorus	528.3 mg

Lunch

Deli Chicken Gyros*
2/3 of a steamed medium artichoke without salt dipped in 2 tablespoons light fat mayonnaise mixed with 2 tablespoons of balsamic vinegar
1/8 cup canned mandarin oranges (juice packed, drained)
1/3 cup fat-free frozen yogurt with low-calorie sweetener and 3 gingersnap cookies

Calories	656
Calories from Fat	115
Total Fat	12.8 g
Saturated Fat	3.46 g
Trans Fat	0.03 g
Cholesterol	33 mg
Sodium	1049 mg
Potassium	1259 mg
Total Carbohydrate	107 g
Dietary Fiber	17 g
Sugars	41 g
Protein	27 g
Phosphorus	484 mg

Dinner

2 oz broiled lamb chop with 1 tablespoon mint jelly
2/3 cup cooked orzo pasta (fat not added in cooking)
1 small rye roll with 1 tablespoon light margarine with plant sterols
1 1/2 cup steamed broccoli with 1 tablespoon light margarine with plant sterols
Chocolate Dipped Apricots*

Calories	640
Calories from Fat	193
Total Fat	21.4 g
Saturated Fat	7.78 g
Trans Fat	0 g
Cholesterol	48 mg
Sodium	664 mg
Potassium	967 mg
Total Carbohydrate	83 g
Dietary Fiber	12.5 g
Sugars	24.6 g
Protein	32 g
Phosphorus	392 mg

DAY 5 total nutritional value

Calories	1758	**Cholesterol**	91.5 mg	**Total Carbohydrate**	266 g
Calories from Fat	394.2	**Sodium**	2029 mg	Dietary Fiber	36.5 g
Total Fat	43.8 g	**Potassium**	3407 mg	Sugars	102.3 g
Saturated Fat	13.2 g			**Protein**	81 g
Trans Fat	0.03 g			**Phosphorus**	1404 mg

Day 1

2,000 Calories

Breakfast

1 cup plain shredded wheat +
  1/4 cup low-fat granola
1 cup fresh raspberries, 1 cup
  honeydew melon balls
1 cup 1% milk
1/2 cup vegetable juice (low
  sodium)
8 pecan halves

Calories	612
Calories from Fat	127
Total Fat	14.1 g
Saturated Fat	2.85 g
Trans Fat	0 g
Cholesterol	12 mg
Sodium	294 mg
Potassium	1494 mg
Total Carbohydrate	112 g
Dietary Fiber	19 g
Sugars	46 g
Protein	20.5 g
Phosphorus	593 mg

Lunch

Sandwich made with 2 large
  slices toasted Pumpernickel
  bread (1.5 oz each), 1 medium
  tomato (sliced), 2 romaine
  lettuce leaves, 1/2 cup sprouts,
  3 oz tuna fish (canned in water
  without salt, drained) mixed
  with 1/2 cup water chestnuts,
  and 1 tablespoon reduced fat
  mayonnaise
1 cup 1% milk
Blackberry Fool* + 3/8 cup extra
  Blackberries as garnish
10 peanuts (no salt)

Calories	718
Calories from Fat	149.4
Total Fat	16.6 g
Saturated Fat	4.2 g
Trans Fat	0 g
Cholesterol	51.6 mg
Sodium	945 mg
Potassium	1414 mg
Total Carbohydrate	101 g
Dietary Fiber	15.4 g
Sugars	34 g
Protein	44.5 g
Phosphorus	741 mg

Dinner

Pork Loin Chops with Mushroom
  Sauce*
1/2 cup mashed potatoes with
  1 teaspoon light margarine with
  plant stanols
1 oz (100%) whole-wheat dinner roll
1 cup unsweetened applesauce
1 1/2 cups steamed broccoli (no
  salt) with 2 teaspoons light
  margarine with plant stanols

Calories	650
Calories from Fat	178
Total Fat	19.8 g
Saturated Fat	5.3 g
Trans Fat	0 g
Cholesterol	60 mg
Sodium	767 mg
Potassium	1672 mg
Total Carbohydrate	86 g
Dietary Fiber	16.4 g
Sugars	32 g
Protein	36.7 g
Phosphorus	490.5 mg

DAY 1 total nutritional value

Calories	1980	**Cholesterol**	123.8 mg	**Total Carbohydrate**	299 g
Calories from Fat	455	**Sodium**	2005 mg	Dietary Fiber	51 g
Total Fat	50.6 g	**Potassium**	4580 mg	Sugars	112 g
Saturated Fat	12.4 g			**Protein**	102 g
Trans Fat	0 g			**Phosphorus**	1824 mg

Day 2

2,000 Calories

Breakfast

(3 oz) cranberry nut muffin or loaf
Banana medium (8 oz)
8 oz skim milk
Omelet made with 2 large egg
    whites and 1/2 cup raw green
    peppers and 1/2 cup onions
    sautéed with 1/2 tablespoon
    light margarine with plant
    sterols

Calories	717
Calories from Fat	180
Total Fat	20 g
Saturated Fat	4.2 g
Trans Fat	0 g
Cholesterol	38.9 mg
Sodium	527 mg
Potassium	1581 mg
Total Carbohydrate	116 g
Dietary Fiber	9.5 g
Sugars	68 g
Protein	24 g
Phosphorus	446 mg

Lunch

2 servings of Brown Rice and
    Edamame Salad*
1 1/4 cups watermelon balls
6 oz plain skim milk yogurt
1 cup cooked Brussels sprouts
    (no salt) with 4 walnut halves
    chopped

Calories	641
Calories from Fat	149
Total Fat	16.6 g
Saturated Fat	2 g
Trans Fat	0 g
Cholesterol	83 mg
Sodium	556 mg
Potassium	1825 mg
Total Carbohydrate	101 g
Dietary Fiber	18 g
Sugars	38 g
Protein	32 g
Phosphorus	704 mg

Dinner

1 serving Chicken and Almond
    Stew*
2 oz rye bread with
    1 1/2 tablespoons light
    margarine with plant sterols
3/4 cup fresh pineapple chunks +
    1 1/4 cup fresh strawberries
1 cup steamed green beans (from
    fresh, no salt or fat added)

Calories	630
Calories from Fat	164
Total Fat	18.2 g
Saturated Fat	3.8 g
Trans Fat	0 g
Cholesterol	40 mg
Sodium	1094 mg
Potassium	1499 mg
Total Carbohydrate	88 g
Dietary Fiber	20 g
Sugars	30 g
Protein	33 g
Phosphorus	486 mg

DAY 2 total nutritional value

Calories	1989	**Cholesterol**	162 mg	**Total Carbohydrate**	306 g
Calories from Fat	493	**Sodium**	2177 mg	Dietary Fiber	48 g
Total Fat	54.8 g	**Potassium**	4905 mg	Sugars	136 g
Saturated Fat	10 g			**Protein**	88 g
Trans Fat	0 g			**Phosphorus**	1635 mg

Day 3

2,000 Calories

Breakfast

1 cup plain spoon-sized shredded wheat with 2 tablespoons dried sweetened cranberries and 1 cup 1% milk

1 oz slice unfrosted raisin bread with 1 tablespoon cashew butter without salt and 1 teaspoon light jam

Calories	572
Calories from Fat	116.1
Total Fat	12.9 g
Saturated Fat	3.6 g
Trans Fat	0 g
Cholesterol	12 mg
Sodium	235 mg
Potassium	965 mg
Total Carbohydrate	105 g
Dietary Fiber	11.5 g
Sugars	38.5 g
Protein	20 g
Phosphorus	555 mg

Lunch

1 serving Black Bean Tacos*

1/2 cup brown rice (long grain without salt)

3 1/2 oz peeled, sliced ripe plantain with 1/2 teaspoon canola oil on top (bake in 450 degree oven until brown turning once, should take about 10 min.)

6 oz non-fat yogurt (plain) shared between the tacos and the plantains

Salad made with 1 cup romaine lettuce shredded, 1/4 cup chopped cilantro, 3/4 cup raw tomato, 3/4 cup raw cucumber, 2 oz low-fat cheddar cheese, 1 tablespoon avocado, and 1 tablespoon fat-free ranch dressing

Calories	710
Calories from Fat	138.6
Total Fat	15.4 g
Saturated Fat	4.3 g
Trans Fat	0 g
Cholesterol	16 mg
Sodium	1017 mg
Potassium	2137 mg
Total Carbohydrate	113 g
Dietary Fiber	14 g
Sugars	41 g
Protein	38 g
Phosphorus	957 mg

Dinner

1 serving Miso Salmon*

2/3 cup cooked quinoa mixed with 1/2 cup corn (corn is frozen)

1 1/4 cups Crenshaw melon mixed with 1 kiwi

1 cup raw zucchini, 1 cup snow peas, 1 cup sliced red bell pepper sautéed with 1 1/2 tablespoons light margarine with plant stanols

Calories	685
Calories from Fat	
Total Fat	21.6 g
Saturated Fat	4.3 g
Trans Fat	0 g
Cholesterol	80 mg
Sodium	609 mg
Potassium	1970 mg
Total Carbohydrate	83 g
Dietary Fiber	15 g
Sugars	32 g
Protein	41 g
Phosphorus	640 mg

DAY 3 total nutritional value

Calories	1967	**Cholesterol**	109 mg	**Total Carbohydrate**	301 g
Calories from Fat	449.1	**Sodium**	1862 mg	Dietary Fiber	41 g
Total Fat	49.9 g	**Potassium**	5072 mg	Sugars	111 g
Saturated Fat	12.3 g			**Protein**	99 g
Trans Fat	0 g			**Phosphorus**	2152 mg

Day 4
2,000 Calories

Breakfast

1 1/2 cups raisin bran with 1 cup
  1% milk
8 oz raw apple cut up with
  8 walnut halves

Calories	615
Calories from Fat	138
Total Fat	15.3 g
Saturated Fat	2.9 g
Trans Fat	0 g
Cholesterol	12 mg
Sodium	485 mg
Potassium	1161 mg
Total Carbohydrate	115 g
Dietary Fiber	18.7 g
Sugars	65 g
Protein	18.5 g
Phosphorus	666 mg

Lunch

Ravioli, Asparagus and Cherry
  Tomato Salad*
2 oz buffalo burger, 1 cup
  mushrooms cooked in
  1 tablespoon light margarine
  with plant stanols, 1 leaf Bibb
  lettuce, 100% whole wheat
  hamburger bun (2 oz)
2/3 cup fat-free frozen yogurt
  with 3/4 cup blueberries on top

Calories	677
Calories from Fat	196
Total Fat	21.8 g
Saturated Fat	7.7 g
Trans Fat	0 g
Cholesterol	81 mg
Sodium	741 mg
Potassium	1264 mg
Total Carbohydrate	93 g
Dietary Fiber	10.7 g
Sugars	45 g
Protein	34.6 g
Phosphorus	539 mg

Dinner

Seared Chicken with Winter
  Squash Sauce*
7 1/2 oz baked potato with skin
  (no salt added), 1 tablespoon
  light margarine with stanols,
  1 tablespoon fat-free sour cream
1 cup cubed papaya + 17 red
  grapes
2 cups raw broccoflower
  (steamed without fat or salt),
  1/2 tablespoon light margarine
  with stanols

Calories	695
Calories from Fat	76.5
Total Fat	8.5 g
Saturated Fat	4.7 g
Trans Fat	0 g
Cholesterol	81 mg
Sodium	633 mg
Potassium	2479 mg
Total Carbohydrate	96 g
Dietary Fiber	14.1 g
Sugars	31 g
Protein	42 g
Phosphorus	554 mg

DAY 4 total nutritional value

Calories	1987	**Cholesterol**	175 mg	**Total Carbohydrate**	304 g
Calories from Fat	410	**Sodium**	1859 mg	Dietary Fiber	43.5 g
Total Fat	45.6 g	**Potassium**	4904 mg	Sugars	141 g
Saturated Fat	15.3 g			**Protein**	95 g
Trans Fat	0 g			**Phosphorus**	1758 mg

Day 5
2,000 Calories

Breakfast

2 slices 7 grain toast with
  1 tablespoon light margarine
  with stanols
1/2 cup sweet potato fries (oven
  baked with 1 teaspoon canola
  oil no salt added)
1 cup 1% milk
Omelet or scramble made with
  1/4 cup low-cholesterol egg
  substitute (from frozen), 1 oz
  low-fat cheddar cheese, 1/4 cup
  tomatoes (drained), 1/4 cup
  mushrooms, 1/4 cup roasted
  asparagus (made from 1/2 cup
  fresh) all no salt added
2 small plums, 1 (6 OZ) white
  peach

Calories	742
Calories from Fat	
Total Fat	24.3 g
Saturated Fat	6.4 g
Trans Fat	0 g
Cholesterol	19 mg
Sodium	751 mg
Potassium	1835 mg
Total Carbohydrate	98 g
Dietary Fiber	12.8 g
Sugars	57 g
Protein	36.7 g
Phosphorus	712 mg

Lunch

Stuffed Tomatoes with Tabouli*
Chickpea, green pea, corn, and
  carrot salad (mix together
  1/2 cup chickpeas [no fat
  added], 1/2 cup chopped
  carrots, 1/8 cup green peas
  and corn [from frozen],
  2 dates cut up in small pieces,
  3 tablespoons 2 fresh mint
  leaves, 1 teaspoon olive oil,
  2 tablespoon lemon juice,
  1/8 teaspoon cumin seeds, dash
  of nutmeg) on 2 outer leafs of
  lettuce
1 oz whole-wheat pita bread
6 oz plain non-fat yogurt
2 fresh apricots, 6 fresh cherries

Calories	705
Calories from Fat	
Total Fat	14.4 g
Saturated Fat	2.2 g
Trans Fat	0 g
Cholesterol	13.4 mg
Sodium	997 mg
Potassium	2118 mg
Total Carbohydrate	117 g
Dietary Fiber	21.5 g
Sugars	54 g
Protein	36 g
Phosphorus	709 mg

Dinner

Spaghetti Squash with sauce
  and cheese with 2 cups
  squash (baked no salt),
  (1/2 cup spaghetti sauce [low-
  sodium] pureed with 1/2 cup
  carrots [from frozen], 1/4 cup
  cooked zucchini, and 1/4 cup
  mushrooms), 2 tablespoons
  low-sodium Parmesan Cheese
Broccoli salad with 1 cup raw
  broccoli, 2 1/2 tablespoons
  dried sweetened cranberries,
  1 teaspoon olive oil mixed with
  3 tablespoon Apple cider
  vinegar, 10 peanuts
1 egg dinner roll (1 oz)
Old Fashioned Ice Cream Soda*

Calories	548
Calories from Fat	
Total Fat	16.6 g
Saturated Fat	4.6 g
Trans Fat	0 g
Cholesterol	25 mg
Sodium	408 mg
Potassium	1548 mg
Total Carbohydrate	89 g
Dietary Fiber	16.6 g
Sugars	44 g
Protein	18 g
Phosphorus	400 mg

DAY 5 total nutritional value

Calories	1996	**Cholesterol**	57 mg	**Total Carbohydrate**	304 g
Calories from Fat		**Sodium**	2155 mg	Dietary Fiber	51 g
Total Fat	55 g	**Potassium**	5501 mg	Sugars	155 g
Saturated Fat	13.2 g			**Protein**	91 g
Trans Fat	0 g			**Phosphorus**	1822 mg

Alphabetical Index

Subject Index